THE HEALING ENEMA COOKBOOK

50+ Enema Recipes to Promote Health and Well-being

ELIZABETH MORGAN

AUTHOR'S NOTE

This book is written for you. It is my great joy to experience the benefits of improved health and well-being. Now, I want everybody to have an opportunity to share in it.

At one point in my life I would have not even wanted to hear about an enema. Six years ago, I was facing several health conditions and began making intentional changes to my lifestyle. I discovered enemas with therapeutic benefits and they quickly became a regular part of my routine.

As a result of what I call Healing Enemas and other practices that eliminate toxins, reduce inflammation and support liver and other vital organs, I am healthier than I may have ever been as an adult. And I look and feel years younger.

If you know me, you will now know what I mean when I talk about my morning coffee or tea!

I sincerely wish you the same success and improved health!

Elizabeth Morgan

www.healingenema.com

FOR YOUR INFORMATION

The content of The Healing Enema Cookbook is does not equal medical advice.

The information in this book is not meant to diagnose, treat or cure any illness, sickness or disease. Please consult your physician before you try any of these cleansing protocols. All information in this enema collection is purely for research and informational purposes only. Follow any of these cleansing protocol procedures at your own risk.

There are many practices, including Healing Enemas, that one can do to maintain, improve, and treat their own health. There are times when medical advice and treatment should be pursued. Please use your judgement in this wisely.

Links to recommended products are for your reference and convenience. Some links will provide additional income to support this book.

THE HEALING ENEMA

A Healing Enema is the placement of a prepared solution into the lower bowel for the purpose of improving health and well-being by cleansing, detoxification and replenishment.

BENEFITS OF A HEALING ENEMA

Whatever type of enema you apply it will help clean the colon. There are many benefits of maintaining a clean colon. Some of them are:

- The regular clearing of the bowels helps the digestive system work more efficiently.
- Constipation is prevented and there is a reduction in related conditions like hemorrhoids and inflamed veins.
- Many feel an increased energy as the toxins in the bowels are regularly released.
- Nutrients are absorbed better in the colon because the mucus buildup is removed.
- There is a reduced risk of cancer since toxins and carcinogens are removed from the body.
- Body functions will be more efficiently maintained.

Healing enemas can be divided into three categories: Retention Enemas, Implant Enemas and Cleansing Enemas.

CLEANSING ENEMA

A Cleansing Enema is usually made of at least one quart of water and the additives have cleansing properties. It is not intended to be held in the bowel but instead to flush out obstructions and accumulated waste.

A Cleansing Enema is often given before the retention and implant enemas as part of an enema stack. Stacking enemas can contribute to effectiveness of the treatments.

RETENTION ENEMA

A Retention Enema is held in the bowel for fifteen minutes or longer allowing the solution to pass through membranes into the system. One of the most popular retention enemas is the Coffee Enema.

IMPLANT ENEMA

An Implant Enema consists of a smaller amount of water and a beneficial additive that is held in the bowel for 45 minutes and often overnight. The liquid and nutrients are totally absorbed into the body.

THE CLEANSING ENEMA

A cleansing enema is given to relieve constipation or to cleanse the bowel before a retention enema, enema implant or medical procedure.

The cleansing enema is only held in the bowel until you feel the natural urge to eliminate the water and the loose fecal material. It is used to gently flush waste out of the colon.

Over time the colon walls become encrusted with non-eliminated toxins and waste, making it sluggish, inefficient and sometimes sick. An average person may have up to 10 pounds or more of non-eliminated waste in the large intestine.

HOW TO ADMINISTER THE CLEANSING ENEMA

The best position to assume when receiving the Cleansing Enema is on your back with your hips slightly raised. After the enema has been inserted, continue to lay on your back with your knees to your chest holding the solution in your body for as long as you can before releasing it. Do not roll from side to side.

. . .

If you do not feel the urge to expel the liquid, simply stand up and move around as usual until you do. Sometimes the enema will not be entirely evacuated because of poor hydration. The body has absorbed the water and nutrients to replenish itself.

HEALTH NOTE

All information in this enema collection is purely for research and informational purposes only. Follow any of these cleansing protocol procedures at your own risk.

GENTLE CLEANSING ENEMA

The gentlest, safest cleansing enema is simply warm filtered water inserted and held for as long as possible.

PREPARE THE GENTLE CLEANSING ENEMA

Ingredients:

2+ cups Filtered Water

Steps:

- Heat the filtered water to slightly warmer than your body
- Add the warm water to an enema bag
- Administer the enema or bucket

WHY FILTERED WATER?

Tap water contains chlorine and other additives that are harmful to your gut flora.

ADMINISTER THE GENTLE CLEANSING ENEMA

The best position to assume when receiving the Gentle Cleansing Enema is on your back with your hips slightly raised. Slowly insert the enema tip and apply as much of the enema solution as you can hold. After the enema has been inserted, continue to lay on your back with your knees to your chest holding the solution in your body for as long as you can before releasing it. Do not roll from side to side.

If you do not feel the urge to expel the liquid, simply stand up and move around as usual until you do. Sometimes the enema will not be entirely evacuated because of poor hydration. The body has absorbed the water and nutrients to its benefit.

APPLE CIDER VINEGAR ENEMA

An Apple Cider Vinegar Enema (ACV) is one of the oldest recorded enemas. It helps fortify the body with vitamins and minerals and offers a long list of health and wellness benefits.

BENEFITS OF APPLE CIDER VINEGAR ENEMAS

- Apple Cider Vinegar Enemas deliver over forty vitamins and minerals.
- Apple Cider Vinegar Enemas help balance pH in the body.
- They create a more alkaline environment that helps eliminate Candida and yeast infections.
- Apple Cider Vinegar Enemas are effective in treating high blood pressure and high cholesterol.
- Apple Cider Vinegar Enemas help with insomnia and fatigue.
- Apple Cider Vinegar Enemas assist in the detoxification of the liver and kidneys.
- Apple Cider Vinegar Enemas help control asthma.
- Apple Cider Vinegar Enemas contribute to good skin health.

PREPARE THE APPLE CIDER VINEGAR ENEMA SOLUTION

Ingredients:

1 - 4 Tbsp of Organic Apple Cider Vinegar
2+ cups Filtered Water

Steps:

1. Heat the filtered water to slightly warmer than your body
2. Add the Organic Apple Cider Vinegar and stir
3. Add the solution to the enema bag or bucket
4. Administer the enema

ADMINISTER THE APPLE CIDER VINEGAR ENEMA

The best position to assume when receiving the Apple Cider Vinegar Enema is on your back with your hips slightly raised. Slowly insert the enema tip and apply as much of the enema solution as you can hold. After the enema has been inserted, continue to lay on your back with your knees to your chest holding the solution in your body for as long as you can before releasing it. Do not roll from side to side.

If you do not feel the urge to expel the liquid, simply stand up and move around as usual until you do. Sometimes the enema will not be entirely evacuated because of poor hydration. The body has absorbed the water and nutrients to its benefit.

THE APPLE CIDER VINEGAR ENEMA CAN HELP

Asthma
Candida
Congestion
Detoxification
Fatigue

High Blood Pressure
High Cholesterol
Insomnia
Liver Support
Mineral Deficiency
Skin Rejuvenation
Viral Infections
Vitamin Deficiency
Yeast Infections

EPSOM SALT ENEMA

Epsom Salts Enemas are used for the relief of muscle aches and pains and for relief from constipation.

BENEFITS OF THE EPSOM SALT ENEMA

Using Epsom salts in an enema is a faster and safer way to achieve effects than when taking the salts orally.

- Epsom Salt Enemas can help stabilize moods.
- They help relieve stress, anxiety and depression.
- Epsom Salt Enemas help relax muscles and relieve muscle pain.
- Epsom Salt Enemas reduce inflammation in internal organs.
- Epsom Salt Enemas improves symptoms of chronic fatigue.
- Epsom Salt Enemas boost the immune system.
- Epsom Salt Enemas help improve the body's natural detoxification process.
- Epsom Salt Enemas promote natural healing process.
- Epsom Salt Enemas help relax bowel muscles and relieving constipation.

PREPARE THE EPSOM SALT ENEMA SOLUTION

Ingredients:

4 Tbsp Epsom Salts
2+ cups Filtered Water

Steps:

1. Heat the filtered water to slightly warmer than your body
2. Add the Epsom Salts to warm water and mix until salt is dissolved
3. Add the solution to the enema bag or bucket
4. Administer the enema

* Only use Epsom Salts that has been tested for human use.

ADMINISTER THE APPLE CIDER VINEGAR ENEMA

The best position to assume when receiving the Epsom Salts Enema is on your back with your hips slightly raised. Slowly insert the enema tip and apply as much of the enema solution as you can hold. After the enema has been inserted, continue to lay on your back with your knees to your chest holding the solution in your body for as long as you can before releasing it. Do not roll from side to side.

If you do not feel the urge to expel the liquid, simply stand up and move around as usual until you do. Sometimes the enema will not be entirely evacuated because of poor hydration. The body has absorbed the water and nutrients to its benefit.

CAUTIONS AND CONSIDERATIONS:

Do not administer an Epsom Salts Enema if you have stomach pain, nausea, or vomiting.

It is dangerous to ingest too much Epsom Salts. Do not take more than the recommended amount.

THE EPSOM SALTS ENEMA CAN HELP

Anxiety
Cardiovascular Disease
Chronic Fatigue
Constipation
Depression
Detoxification
Immune System Support
Improved Bowel Function
Inflammation
Muscle Pain

SALT WATER ENEMA

A salt water enema is the most comfortable enemas. If you are doing enema for the first time, the salt water enema is the best choice.

BENEFITS OF SALT WATER ENEMAS

A Salt Water Enema is very effective for softening old, impacted feces that is clogging a colon. This enema does not draw electrolytes from the body. Because it does not draw water into the colon it is a good enema when a longer retention is desired.

- Salt Water Enemas improve metabolism that can lead to weight loss.
- Salt Water Enemas remove accumulated waste in the colon.
- They add essential minerals and nutrients to the body.

PREPARE THE SALT WATER ENEMA SOLUTION

Ingredients:

2 tsp pure Sea Salt

2+ cups Filtered Water

Steps:

1. Heat the filtered water to slightly warmer than your body
2. Add the sea salt to the 2+ cups warm water
3. Mix well until all salt is dissolved
4. Add the solution to the enema bag or bucket
5. Administer the enema

ADMINISTER THE SALT WATER ENEMA

The best position to assume when receiving the Salt Water Enema is on your back with your hips slightly raised. Slowly insert the enema tip and apply as much of the enema solution as you can hold. After the enema has been inserted, continue to lay on your back with your knees to your chest holding the solution in your body for as long as you can before releasing it. Do not roll from side to side.

If you do not feel the urge to expel the liquid, simply stand up and move around as usual until you do. Sometimes the enema will not be entirely evacuated because of poor hydration. The body has absorbed the water and nutrients to its benefit.

THE SALT WATER ENEMA CAN HELP

Constipation
Chronic fatigue
Cramping and Abdominal Pains
Allergies
Suspected Cancers
Irritable Bowel Syndrome
Parasites

SUPER COLON CLEANSING ENEMA

BENEFITS OF THE SUPER COLON CLEANSING ENEMA

This Super Colon Cleansing Enema is a combination of ingredients that work well individually. Taken together they clean the colon and stimulate the liver to release bile, contribute to gut health and carry toxins from the body.

- Super Colon Cleansing Enemas are a good blood purifier.
- They help balance the bacteria in the gut.
- Super Colon Cleansing Enemas help with Leaky Gut Syndrome.
- They enhance cleansing effects in the colon.
- Super Colon Cleansing Enemas provide support for the liver.
- They replenish minerals in the body.
- Super Colon Cleansing Enemas can help heal yeast infections.
- Super Colon Cleansing Enemas contribute to increased energy.
- They are an effective part of a detoxification plan.

PREPARE THE SUPER COLON CLEANSING ENEMA SOLUTION

Ingredients:

6 Chlorophyll Capsules
1 - 2 capsules Probiotic Formula, therapeutic strength
1 - 2 teaspoons Bentonite Clay powder
2+ cups Filtered Water

Steps:

1. Heat the filtered water to slightly warmer than your body
2. Empty Chlorophyll Capsules and Probiotic into water in a glass jar
3. Add Bentonite Clay Powder
4. Stir with wooden spoon* or shake until dissolved
5. Add the solution to the enema bag or bucket
6. Administer the enema

* Use a wooden spoon to stir because the Bentonite Clay will attract metals from another type of spoon and release these toxins into your body.

ADMINISTER THE SUPER COLON CLEANSING ENEMA

The best position to assume when receiving the Super Colon Cleansing Enema is on your back with your hips slightly raised. Slowly insert the enema tip and apply as much of the enema solution as you can hold. After the enema has been inserted, continue to lay on your back with your knees to your chest holding the solution in your body for as long as you can before releasing it. Do not roll from side to side.

If you do not feel the urge to expel the liquid, simply stand up and move around as usual until you do. Sometimes the enema will not be entirely evacuated because of poor hydration. The body has absorbed the water and nutrients to its benefit.

THE SUPER COLON CLEANSING ENEMA CAN HELP

Allergy Relief
Blood Purifier
Colon Cleanse
Complexion
Detoxification
Fatigue
Gut Bacteria Balance
Leaky Gut Syndrome
Liver Support
Mineral Deficiency
Yeast Infections

RETENTION ENEMAS

A Retention Enema is held in the bowel for fifteen minutes or longer allowing the solution to pass through membranes into the system. One of the most popular Retention Enemas is the Coffee Enema.

HOW TO ADMINISTER THE RETENTION ENEMA

The best position to assume when receiving Retention Enemas is on your back with your hips slightly raised. After the enema has been inserted, roll onto your right side and hold the solution inside for fifteen to 45 minutes before expelling it. Do not roll from side to side.

If you do not feel the urge to expel the liquid, simply stand up and move around as usual until you do. Sometimes the enema will not be evacuated because of poor hydration. The body has absorbed the water and nutrients to its benefit.

HEALTH NOTE

All information in this enema collection is purely for research and informational purposes only. Follow any of these cleansing protocol procedures at your own risk.

AGRIMONY ENEMA

BENEFITS OF AGRIMONY ENEMAS

- Agrimony Enemas help dispel gas.
- Agrimony Enemas are helpful with diarrhea.
- They help remove mucus.
- Agrimony Enemas can treat symptoms of colitis.
- Agrimony Enemas are used to manage incontinence,
- They are used for healing the body's membranes.

PREPARE THE AGRIMONY ENEMA SOLUTION

Ingredients:

I Dose Agrimony Extract
Filtered Water

Steps:

1. Heat 1 - 2 cups water to slightly warmer than your body

2. Stir 1 dose Agrimony Extract into the water
3. Add the solution to the enema bag or bucket
4. Administer the enema

ADMINISTER THE AGRIMONY ENEMA

The best position to assume when receiving the Agrimony Enema Implant is on your back with your hips slightly raised. After the enema has been inserted, roll onto your right side and hold the liquid inside up to 45 minutes before releasing it. Do not roll from side to side.

Some people claim benefits to holding the liquids long enough for them to be fully absorbed by the body. This is easily achieved by administering the Agrimony Enema Implant before going to sleep.

THE AGRIMONY ENEMA CAN HELP

Colitis
Colon Cleanse
Diarrhea
Gas
Healing
Incontinence

ALOE VERA ENEMA

Aloe Vera Enemas are soothing with strong anti-inflammatory properties.

BENEFITS OF ALOE VERA ENEMAS

- Aloe Vera Enemas have strong anti-inflammatory properties.
- An aloe vera enema is good for those suffering from hemorrhoids.
- Aloe Vera Enemas can help stop bleeding associated with hemorrhoids.
- Aloe Vera Enemas can help in the healing of hemorrhoids.
- They promote healing of the intestinal tract.
- Aloe Vera Enemas are helpful inn treatment of irritable bowel syndrome or diverticulitis.

PREPARE THE ALOE VERA ENEMA SOLUTION

Ingredients:

1/3 to ½ cup Aloe Vera Juice
Filtered Water

Steps:

1. Heat 2 - 4 cups water to slightly warmer than your body
2. Combine the Aloe Vera Juice and the water
3. Add the solution to the enema bag or bucket
4. Administer the enema

ADMINISTER THE ALOE VERA ENEMA

The best position to assume when receiving the Aloe Vera Enema is on your back with your hips slightly raised. After the enema has been inserted, roll onto your right side and hold the solution inside for fifteen minutes to 45 minutes before expelling it. Do not roll from side to side.

If you do not feel the urge to expel the liquid, simply stand up and move around as usual until you do. Sometimes the enema will not be evacuated because of poor hydration. The body has absorbed the water and nutrients to its benefit.

THE ALOE VERA ENEMA CAN HELP

Inflammation
Hemorrhoids
Irritable Bowel Syndrome
Diverticulitis.

ANISEED BASIL ENEMA

An Aniseed Basil Enema is both calming and refreshing. It stimulates circulation and is cleansing.

BENEFITS OF ANISEED BASIL ENEMAS

- Aniseed Basil Enemas stimulate circulation and cleansing.
- Aniseed Basil Enemas introduce several important micronutrients to the body.
- Aniseed Basil Enemas contribute to decreased symptoms of mild to moderate depression.
- Aniseed Basil Enemas can help prevent bone loss and protect against osteoporosis.
- Aniseed Basil Enemas help reduce high blood sugar levels.
- Aniseed Basil Enemas are high in antioxidants.
- Aniseed Basil Enemas supports healthy liver function.
- They are effective in detoxification.
- Aniseed Basil Enemas promote a healthy gut.
- Aniseed Basil Enemas may help fight cancer.
- Aniseed Basil Enemas are natural antibacterial agents.
- They are a natural adaptogen.

PREPARE THE ANISEED BASIL ENEMA SOLUTION

Ingredients:

1 tsp Aniseed Extract
20 drops Basil Extract
Filtered Water

Steps:

1. Heat 1 - 2 cups water to slightly warmer than your body
2. Stir Aniseed and Basil Extracts into the water
3. Add the solution to the enema bag or bucket
4. Administer the enema

ADMINISTER THE ANISEED BASIL ENEMA

The best position to assume when receiving the Aniseed Basil Enema Implant is on your back with your hips slightly raised. After the enema has been inserted, roll onto your right side and hold the liquid inside up to 45 minutes before releasing it. Do not roll from side to side.

Some people claim benefits to holding the liquids long enough for them to be fully absorbed by the body. This is easily achieved by administering the Aniseed Basil Enema Implant before going to sleep.

THE ANISEED BASIL ENEMA CAN HELP

Adaptogen
Antibacterial
Cancer
Colon Cleansing
Circulation

Depression
High Blood Sugar
Inflammation
Liver Health
Nutritional Deficiencies
Bone Health

ANISEED FENNEL ENEMA

BENEFITS OF ANISEED-FENNEL ENEMAS

- Aniseed Fennel Enemas stimulate circulation and cleansing.
- They introduce several important micronutrients to the body.
- Aniseed Fennel Enemas contribute to decreased symptoms of depression.
- Aniseed Fennel Enemas can help prevent bone loss.
- Aniseed Fennel Enemas help reduce high blood sugar levels.
- They support the blood and circulatory system.
- Aniseed Fennel Enemas are high in antioxidants.
- They can help regulate blood pressure.
- Aniseed Fennel Enemas can help improve eyesight.
- Aniseed Fennel Enemas can help manage blood sugar levels.

PREPARE THE ANISEED FENNEL ENEMA SOLUTION

Ingredients:

1 tsp Aniseed Extract

20 drops Fennel Extract
Filtered Water

Steps:

1. Heat 2 - 4 cups water to slightly warmer than your body
2. Stir Aniseed and Fennel Extracts into the water
3. Add the solution to the enema bag or bucket
4. Administer the enema

ADMINISTER THE ANISEED FENNEL ENEMA

The best position to assume when receiving the Aniseed Fennel Enema Implant is on your back with your hips slightly raised. After the enema has been inserted, roll onto your right side and hold the liquid inside up to 45 minutes before releasing it. Do not roll from side to side.

Some people claim benefits to holding the liquids long enough for them to be fully absorbed by the body. This is easily achieved by administering the Aniseed Fennel Enema Implant before going to sleep.

THE ANISEED FENNEL ENEMA CAN HELP

Asthma
Bone Health
Blood Pressure
Blood Purification
Cancer
Colon Cleansing
Constipation
Circulation
Depression
Eyesight

Heart Health
High Blood Sugar
Indigestion
Immunity
Inflammation
Irritable Bowel Syndrome
Metabolism
Nutritional Deficiencies
Skin Rejuvenation

BENTONITE ENEMA

The Bentonite Enema works by collecting and removing toxins and harmful material rather than absorption by the body.

BENEFITS OF BENTONITE ENEMAS

- Bentonite Enemas improve intestinal regularity.
- Bentonite Enemas provide relief from chronic constipation, diarrhea, indigestion and ulcers.
- Bentonite Enemas result in a surge in physical energy.
- Bentonite Enemas contribute to a clearer complexion.
- Bentonite Enemas leads to brighter, whiter eyes.
- Bentonite Enemas may enhance alertness.
- Bentonite Enemas may result in an emotional uplift.
- Bentonite Enemas improve tissue and gum repair.
- Bentonite Enemas may increase resistance to infections.
- Bentonite Enemas are an effective solution in treating acute diarrhea.

PREPARE THE BENTONITE ENEMA SOLUTION

Ingredients:

4 - 6 Oz. Bentonite Clay liquid
Filtered Water

Steps:

1. Heat 2 - 4 cups water to slightly warmer than your body
2. Thoroughly mix Bentonite Clay and warm water
3. Add the solution to the enema bag or bucket
4. Administer the enema

ADMINISTER THE BENTONITE ENEMA

The best position to assume when receiving the Bentonite Enema is on your back with your hips slightly raised. After the enema has been inserted, roll onto your right side and hold the solution inside for fifteen minutes to 45 minutes before expelling it. Do not roll from side to side.

If you do not feel the urge to expel the liquid, simply stand up and move around as usual until you do. Sometimes the enema will not be evacuated because of poor hydration. The body has absorbed the water and nutrients to its benefit.

THE BENTONITE ENEMA CAN HELP

Alertness
Constipation
Diarrhea
Emotional Well-being
Increased Energy

Indigestion
Intestinal regularity
Skin Rejuvenation
Tissue and Gum Health
Ulcers
Vision

BURDOCK ROOT ENEMA

There are many benefits to a Burdock Root Enema and it is usually chosen to support the kidneys, bladder and to break down calcium deposits. It is good for supporting the skin, blood and hair.

BENEFITS OF THE BURDOCK ROOT ENEMA

- Burdock Root has potent anti-inflammatory and antibacterial effects on the human body.
- Burdock root has active ingredients to clear the bloodstream of heavy metals toxins.
- It cleanses the blood and improves circulation to the skin surface with a healing effect on acne, eczema, psoriasis and other skin disorders.
- It strengthens the lymphatic system and supports good liver health.
- Burdock root is rich in potassium salts and contains phenolic acids, quercetin and luteolin, which are strong, health-promoting antioxidants.
- Burdock root is a natural diuretic.
- Burdock root contains inulin, a soluble and prebiotic fiber that

helps improve digestion and lower blood sugar, decreasing the severity of diabetic complications.
- Burdock root is a powerful anti-inflammatory, even helping to soothe arthritis.

PREPARE THE BURDOCK ROOT ENEMA SOLUTION

Ingredients:

2 Tbsp chopped Burdock Root
Filtered Water

Steps:

1. Bring 2 Tbsp Burdock Root to a boil in 2 - 4 cups of filtered water
2. Simmer over reduced heat for 15 minutes
3. Strain mixture and dispose of the Burdock root
4. Add water to bring the amount of solution to between 2 - 4 cups
5. Heat or cool to warm, comfortable temperature
6. Add the solution to the enema bag or bucket
7. Administer the enema

ADMINISTER THE BURDOCK ROOT ENEMA

The best position to assume when receiving the Burdock Root Enema is on your back with your hips slightly raised. After the enema has been inserted, roll onto your right side and hold the solution inside for fifteen minutes to 45 minutes before expelling it. Do not roll from side to side.

If you do not feel the urge to expel the liquid, simply stand up and move around as usual until you do. Sometimes the enema will not be evacuated because of poor hydration. The body has absorbed the water and nutrients to its benefit.

THE BURDOCK ROOT ENEMA CAN HELP

Blood Purifier
Calcium Deposits
Circulation Problems
Hair Restoration
Skin Rejuvenation

CASTOR OIL ENEMA

Castor Oil Enemas are used as a laxative, an elixir of youth, and were touted to be a miracle cure for almost every disease on the earth.

BENEFITS OF CASTOR OIL ENEMAS

- Castor Oil Enemas soften stools and relieve constipation.
- Castor Oil Enemas reduce bloating due to gas.
- Castor Oil Enemas are useful in the treatment arthritis and rheumatism.
- Castor Oil Enemas may be helpful in curing sexual disorders.
- Castor Oil Enemas have been effective cure for hyperacidity.
- Castor Oil Enemas can help alleviate back pain.

PREPARE THE CASTOR OIL ENEMA SOLUTION

Ingredients:

1 serving Organic Castor Oil
Filtered Water

Steps:

1. Heat 2 - 4 cups water to slightly warmer than your body
2. Stir 1 serving Organic Castor Oil into the water
3. Add the solution to the enema bag or bucket
4. Administer the enema

ADMINISTER THE CASTOR OIL ENEMA

The best position to assume when receiving the Castor Oil Enema is on your back with your hips slightly raised. After the enema has been inserted, roll onto your right side and hold the solution inside for fifteen minutes to 45 minutes before expelling it. Do not roll from side to side.

If you do not feel the urge to expel the liquid, simply stand up and move around as usual until you do. Sometimes the enema will not be evacuated because of poor hydration. The body has absorbed the water and nutrients to its benefit.

It's a good idea to follow a Castor Oil Enema with a Gentle Cleansing Enema. This will help remove all the traces of oil and prevent leaking oil later.

CAUTIONS AND CONSIDERATIONS

Do not take a castor oil enema if you have the cold or flu, indigestion or diarrhea. Do not take a Castor Oil Enema if you are suffering from Diabetes, obesity or have consumed poison.

THE CASTOR OIL ENEMA CAN HELP

Constipation
Bloating

Arthritis
Rheumatism
Sexual Disorders
pH Balance
Back Pain

CAT'S CLAW ENEMA

Cat's Claw Enemas are known for immune-boosting properties and efficiency in healing intestinal ailments.

BENEFITS OF CAT'S CLAW ENEMAS

- Cat's Claw Enemas can help boost the immune system.
- Cat's Claw Enemas are helpful in the healing of intestinal ailments.
- They cleanse the colon.
- Cat's Claw Enemas aid the healing of bowel disorders such as Chron's, colitis, diverticulitis, leaky gut syndrome and hemorrhoids.
- Cat's Claw Enemas can help reduce intestinal parasites.
- Cat's Claw Enemas aid in restoring friendly bacteria in the colon.

PREPARE THE CAT'S CLAW ENEMA SOLUTION

Ingredients:

2 Tbsp Cat's Claw Powder
Filtered Water

Steps:

1. Bring 2 - 4 cups water to a boil, remove from heat
2. Add 2 Tbsp Cat's Claw powder and let steep for 15 minutes
3. Filter the tea
4. Add water to bring the amount of solution to between 2 - 4 cups
5. Heat or cool to warm, comfortable temperature
6. Add the solution to the enema bag or bucket
7. Administer the enema

ADMINISTER THE CAT'S CLAW ENEMA

The best position to assume when receiving the Cat's Claw Enema is on your back with your hips slightly raised. After the enema has been inserted, roll onto your right side and hold the solution inside for fifteen minutes to 45 minutes before expelling it. Do not roll from side to side.

If you do not feel the urge to expel the liquid, simply stand up and move around as usual until you do. Sometimes the enema will not be evacuated because of poor hydration. The body has absorbed the water and nutrients to its benefit.

THE CAT'S CLAW ENEMA CAN HELP

Chron's
Colitis
Colon Cleansing
Diverticulitis
Gut Bacteria Balance

Hemorrhoids
Immune System
Intestinal Disorders
Intestinal Parasites
Leaky Gut Syndrome

CATNIP TEA ENEMA

The Catnip Tea Enema is very relaxing.

BENEFITS OF CATNIP TEA ENEMAS

- Catnip Tea Enemas soothe and relax the intestinal tract.
- Catnip Tea Enemas help ease pain and cramping in the colon.
- Catnip Tea Enemas can reduce intestinal gas and help relieve constipation.
- Catnip Tea Enemas also help remove mucus from the colon.
- Catnip Tea Enemas are helpful during the cold or flu.
- Catnip Tea Enemas reduce fever quickly and are safe for use in both adults and children.

PREPARE THE CATNIP TEA ENEMA SOLUTION

Ingredients:

2 Tbsp dried Catnip Leaves or 4 Catnip Tea bags
Filtered Water

Steps:

1. Bring 2 - 4 cups water to a boil, remove from heat
2. Add the Catnip Leaves or tea bags and let steep for 15 minutes
3. Strain if needed
4. Add water to bring the amount of solution to between 2 - 4 cups
5. Heat or cool to warm, comfortable temperature
6. Add the solution to the enema bag or bucket
7. Administer the enema

ADMINISTER THE CATNIP TEA ENEMA

The best position to assume when receiving the Catnip Tea Enema is on your back with your hips slightly raised. After the enema has been inserted, roll onto your right side and hold the solution inside for fifteen minutes to 45 minutes before expelling it. Do not roll from side to side.

If you do not feel the urge to expel the liquid, simply stand up and move around as usual until you do. Sometimes the enema will not be evacuated because of poor hydration. The body has absorbed the water and nutrients to its benefit.

THE CATNIP TEA ENEMA CAN HELP

Anti-bacterial
Anti-fungal
Colon Cleanse
Constipation
Cramping
Fever
Gas
Intestinal Tract Problems

CAYENNE ENEMA

Cayenne Enemas are powerfully stimulating without any narcotic effects.

BENEFITS OF CAYENNE ENEMA

- Cayenne Enemas helps regulate blood pressure.
- Cayenne Enemas strengthens the pulse strength.
- Cayenne Enemas helps lower cholesterol.
- Cayenne Enemas helps thin the blood.
- Cayenne Enemas cleans the circulatory system.
- Cayenne Enemas helps heal ulcers.
- Cayenne Enemas can help stop hemorrhaging.
- Cayenne Enemas may speed the healing of wounds.
- Cayenne Enemas helps rebuild damaged tissue.
- Cayenne Enemas ease congestion.
- Cayenne Enemas aids digestions.
- Cayenne Enemas help to regulate bowel movements.
- Cayenne Enemas relieves arthritis and rheumatism.
- Cayenne Enemas prevents the spread of infection.
- Cayenne Enemas relieves and can even numb pain.

PREPARE THE CAYENNE ENEMA SOLUTION

Ingredients:

¼ tsp Cayenne Pepper
Filtered Water

Steps:

1. Heat 2 - 4 cups water to slightly warmer than your body
2. Stir ¼ tsp Cayenne Pepper into the water
3. Add the solution to the enema bag or bucket
4. Administer the enema

ADMINISTER THE CAYENNE ENEMA

The best position to assume when receiving the Cayenne Enema is on your back with your hips slightly raised. After the enema has been inserted, roll onto your right side and hold the solution inside for fifteen minutes to 45 minutes before expelling it. Do not roll from side to side.

If you do not feel the urge to expel the liquid, simply stand up and move around as usual until you do. Sometimes the enema will not be evacuated because of poor hydration. The body has absorbed the water and nutrients to its benefit.

CAUTIONS AND CONSIDERATIONS

The Cayenne Enema will have a burning sensation in the area of the rectum when it comes in contact with tissue. Diluting the solution can help. Preparing the area with a layer of a viscous oil like Castor Oil may offer some protection.

THE CAYENNE ENEMA CAN HELP

Arthritis
Blood Pressure
Cholesterol
Circulation
Congestion
Constipation
Healing
Heart Health
Hemorrhaging
Indigestion
Infection
Pain
Rheumatism
Ulcers

CHAMOMILE ENEMA

Chamomile Enemas are calming and promote relaxation in the body and the digestive system.

BENEFITS OF CHAMOMILE ENEMAS

- Chamomile Enemas promotes relaxation in the body.
- Chamomile Enemas relaxes the digestive system.
- Chamomile Enemas soothes an irritated intestinal tract.
- Chamomile Enemas can reduce abdominal cramps or spasms caused by gas or inflammation.
- Chamomile Enemas may also help relieve hemorrhoids and nausea.
- Chamomile Enemas improve sleep.

PREPARE THE CHAMOMILE ENEMA SOLUTION

Ingredients:

2 Tbsp loose Chamomile or 4 bags of Chamomile Tea

Filtered Water

Steps:

1. Bring 2 - 4 cups water to a boil
2. Remove from heat and add the chamomile
3. Let steep for 15 minutes
4. Strain if needed
5. Add water to bring the amount of solution to between 2 - 4 cups
6. Heat or cool to warm, comfortable temperature
7. Add the solution to the enema bag or bucket
8. Administer the enema

ADMINISTER THE CHAMOMILE ENEMA

The best position to assume when receiving the Chamomile Enema is on your back with your hips slightly raised. After the enema has been inserted, roll onto your right side and hold the solution inside for fifteen minutes to 45 minutes before expelling it. Do not roll from side to side.

If you do not feel the urge to expel the liquid, simply stand up and move around as usual until you do. Sometimes the enema will not be evacuated because of poor hydration. The body has absorbed the water and nutrients to its benefit.

CAUTIONS AND CONSIDERATIONS:

If you have an allergy to ragweed you should not use of chamomile.

Chamomile is a gentle sedative and may cause drowsiness.

THE CHAMOMILE ENEMA CAN HELP

Abdominal Cramps

Digestive system
Gas
Hemorrhoids
Inflammation
Insomnia
Intestinal Irritation
Nausea
Relaxation

COFFEE ENEMA

The Coffee Enema is a powerful retention enema and is useful in the removal of toxins from the body. Coffee Enemas have been shown to reduce the levels of toxicity up to 600%. Coffee Enemas increase the production of Glutathione S-transferase.

The Glutathione enzyme scavenges free radicals that contribute to inflammation, poor gut health, liver disease and damage to cells. Once free radicals are neutralized, bile that is produced from the liver and gallbladder release these substances through bowel movements.

BENEFITS OF THE COFFEE ENEMA

Coffee Enemas have been recorded as early as the late 1800s, but gained popularity when Dr. Max Gerson began using them in his natural treatment of cancer, tuberculosis, and other chronic conditions. According to Max Gerson, "Coffee enemas are not given for the function of the intestines but for the stimulation of the liver."

Here are a Few More Reasons to Try A Coffee Enema:

- Coffee enemas are great pain relievers.
- They clean and heal the colon, improving bowel function.

- Coffee enemas increase energy levels and improve mental clarity.
- They help fight depression, bad moods, sluggishness.
- They help eliminate parasites and candida.
- They relieve frequent constipation, bloating, cramping and nausea.
- Coffee Enemas improve gut health.
- Coffee Enemas detoxifies and helps repair the liver and digestive tissue.
- Coffee Enemas help reduce detoxification reactions during fasting.
- They can help heal chronic health conditions.
- Coffee Enemas are a popular treatments for aid in healing cancer patients.
- They improve blood circulation.
- They contribute to increased immunity.
- They help to promote cellular regeneration.

PREPARE THE COFFEE ENEMA SOLUTION

Ingredients:

3 Tbsp of Organic Coffee
Filtered Water

Steps:

1. Bring 3 Tbsp Organic Coffee to a boil in 2 cups of filtered water.
2. Simmer over reduced heat for 15 minutes.
3. Strain mixture and dispose of the coffee grounds.
4. Add water to bring the amount of solution to between 2 - 4 cups
5. Heat or cool to warm, comfortable temperature
6. Add the solution to the enema bag or bucket

7. Administer the enema

ADMINISTER THE COFFEE ENEMA

The best position to assume when receiving the Coffee Enema is on your back with your hips slightly raised. After the enema has been inserted, roll onto your right side and hold the solution inside for fifteen minutes to 45 minutes before expelling it. Do not roll from side to side.

If you do not feel the urge to expel the liquid, simply stand up and move around as usual until you do. Sometimes the enema will not be evacuated because of poor hydration. The body has absorbed the water and nutrients to its benefit.

THE COFFEE ENEMA CAN HELP

Aging
Blood Purifier
Cancer
Circulation Problems
Constipation
Depression
Detoxification
Fatigue
Focus
Gallbladder Stimulant
Increased Energy
Lack of Concentration
Liver Support
Mental Clarity

DAMIANA ENEMA

The Damiana Enema can be used as a general tonic for the nervous, hormonal, and reproductive systems. Damiana has an ancient reputation as an aphrodisiac and some claim damiana has a relaxing effect similar to low doses of cannabis.

BENEFITS OF THE DAMIANA ENEMA

- The Damiana Enemas helps reduce anxiety.
- The Damiana Enemas can relieve constipation.
- The Damiana Enemas can help with depression.
- The Damiana Enemas can reduce symptoms of erectile dysfunction.
- The Damiana Enemas increases energy.
- They improve bowel function.
- The Damiana Enemas can improve concentration.
- The Damiana Enemas improve problems with menstruation.

PREPARE THE DAMIANA ENEMA SOLUTION

Ingredients:

2 Tbsp organic Damiana Extract Powder
Filtered Water

Steps:

1. Add 2 Tablespoons Damiana Extract Powder to boiling filtered water
2. Simmer over reduced heat for 15 minutes
3. Add water to bring the amount of solution to between 2 - 4 cups
4. Heat or cool to warm, comfortable temperature
5. Add the solution to the enema bag or bucket
6. Administer the enema

ADMINISTER THE DAMIANA ENEMA

The best position to assume when receiving the Damiana Enema is on your back with your hips slightly raised. After the enema has been inserted, roll onto your right side and hold the solution inside for fifteen minutes to 45 minutes before expelling it. Do not roll from side to side.

If you do not feel the urge to expel the liquid, simply stand up and move around as usual until you do. Sometimes the enema will not be evacuated because of poor hydration. The body has absorbed the water and nutrients to its benefit.

DAMIANA ENEMA CAN HELP

Anxiety

Constipation
Depression
Erectile Dysfunction
Fatigue
Improved Bowel Function
Increased Energy
Lack of Concentration
Menstrual Problems

FENUGREEK ENEMA

Fenugreek Enemas are used internally for inflammatory conditions throughout the body.

BENEFITS OF FENUGREEK ENEMAS

- Fenugreek Enemas are used to reduce inflammation.
- Fenugreek Enemas help lubricate and protect mucus membranes in the body.
- Fenugreek Enemas soothe inflammation in the digestive tract.
- Fenugreek Enemas protect against the formation of ulcers in the intestinal tract and relieve pain from existing ulcers.

PREPARE THE FENUGREEK ENEMA SOLUTION

Ingredients:

2 Tbsp Fenugreek Seeds
Filtered Water

Steps:

1. Soak the fenugreek seeds in 2 - 4 cups water overnight
2. Boil the water with the seeds for 5 minutes
3. Remove from heat and strain
4. Add water to bring the amount of solution to between 2 - 4 cups
5. Heat or cool to warm, comfortable temperature
6. Add the solution to the enema bag or bucket
7. Administer the enema

ADMINISTER THE FENUGREEK ENEMA

The best position to assume when receiving the Fenugreek Enema is on your back with your hips slightly raised. After the enema has been inserted, roll onto your right side and hold the solution inside for fifteen minutes to 45 minutes before expelling it. Do not roll from side to side.

If you do not feel the urge to expel the liquid, simply stand up and move around as usual until you do. Sometimes the enema will not be evacuated because of poor hydration. The body has absorbed the water and nutrients to its benefit.

THE FENUGREEK ENEMA CAN HELP

Digestion
Inflammation
Ulcers

FIBER ENEMA

BENEFITS OF FIBER ENEMAS

- The Fiber Enema absorbs toxins and poisons lining the colon wall.
- The Fiber Enema is useful in treatment of fecal incontinence.

PREPARE THE FIBER ENEMA SOLUTION

Ingredients:

2 - 4 Tbsp. Psyllium or (Metamucil)
Filtered Water

Steps:

1. Heat the filtered water to slightly warmer than your body
2. Mix the fiber into 2 cups - 2 quarts warm water
3. You will probably need to keep mixing during the application.
4. Add the solution to the enema bag or bucket

5. Administer the enema

ADMINISTER THE FIBER ENEMA

The best position to assume when receiving the Fiber Enema is on your back with your hips slightly raised. After the enema has been inserted, roll onto your right side and hold the solution inside for fifteen minutes to 45 minutes before expelling it. Do not roll from side to side.

If you do not feel the urge to expel the liquid, simply stand up and move around as usual until you do. Sometimes the enema will not be evacuated because of poor hydration. The body has absorbed the water and nutrients to its benefit.

THE FIBER ENEMA CAN HELP

Detoxification
Fecal Incontinence

FLAXSEED ENEMA

The Flaxseed Enema is soothing and easy to retain.

BENEFITS OF FLAXSEED ENEMAS

- Flaxseed Enemas are antioxidant and help reduce inflammation.
- They contain the essential fatty acid alpha-linolenic acid, also known as ALA.
- Flaxseed Enemas can lower the risk of diabetes.
- Flaxseed Enemas reduce the risk of cancer.
- Flaxseed Enemas can help prevent heart disease.
- Flaxseed Enemas maintain healthy cholesterol levels.
- Flaxseed Enemas are used to manage hunger to reduce weight.
- Flaxseed Enemas help maintain healthy blood sugar levels.

PREPARE THE FLAXSEED ENEMA SOLUTION

Ingredients:

2 Tbsp. Flaxseed Powder
Filtered Water

Steps:

1. Heat 1 - 2 cups water to slightly warmer than your body
2. Stir 2 Tbsp. Flaxseed Powder into the water
3. Add the solution to the enema bag or bucket
4. Administer the enema

ADMINISTER THE FLAXSEED ENEMA

The best position to assume when receiving the Flaxseed Enema Implant is on your back with your hips slightly raised. After the enema has been inserted, roll onto your right side and hold the liquid inside up to 45 minutes before releasing it. Do not roll from side to side.

Some people claim benefits to holding the liquids long enough for them to be fully absorbed by the body. This is easily achieved by administering the Flaxseed Enema Implant before going to sleep.

THE FLAXSEED ENEMA CAN HELP

Blood Sugar
Cancer
Cholesterol
Diabetes
Heart Disease
Hunger Management
Inflammation

Recipe Index

GARLIC ENEMA

Garlic Enemas are more efficient than eating garlic and deliver the benefits directly into the colon.

BENEFITS OF GARLIC ENEMAS

- Garlic Enemas are potent antibiotics and anti-fungal agents.
- Garlic Enemas are an effective anti-parasitic.
- Garlic Enemas are used to eliminate intestinal worms and other parasites.
- Garlic Enemas are used to reduce candida levels in the colon.
- Garlic Enemas relieve symptoms of diarrhea.
- Garlic enemas are helpful in the elimination of toxins and mucus from the colon.
- Garlic Enemas are helpful in reducing fever.

PREPARE THE GARLIC ENEMA SOLUTION

Ingredients:

3 Garlic Cloves
Filtered Water

Steps:

1. Crush the garlic cloves and let them sit for 15 minutes
2. Add the garlic to 2 - 4 cups water
3. Let the mixture sit for at least 2 hours or as long as overnight
4. Strain the mixture
5. Heat the solution to slightly warmer than your body
6. Add the solution to the enema bag or bucket
7. Administer the enema

ADMINISTER THE GARLIC ENEMA

The best position to assume when receiving the Garlic Enema is on your back with your hips slightly raised. After the enema has been inserted, roll onto your right side and hold the solution inside for fifteen minutes to 45 minutes before expelling it. Do not roll from side to side.

If you do not feel the urge to expel the liquid, simply stand up and move around as usual until you do. Sometimes the enema will not be evacuated because of poor hydration. The body has absorbed the water and nutrients to its benefit.

ENEMA STACKING

Follow The Garlic Enema with an Acidophilus Enema or Probiotic Enema to maintain healthy bacteria levels in the colon.

It is also common to combine garlic with an Epsom Salt enema or a Catnip Tea Enema.

CAUTIONS AND CONSIDERATIONS:

If your infection of Candida or Parasites is severe it is best to start with one clove of garlic and gradually increase the strength by adding one clove every day. Do not take more than 4-5 cloves of garlic in a single enema.

If you use Garlic Enemas regularly it may deplete the healthy bacteria in your colon. To add beneficial bacteria back to your colon you can alternate the Garlic Enema with an Acidophilus Enema or Probiotic Enema.

It is normal to feel a warming sensation when applying a Garlic Enema. If the sensation is too strong you can start with a diluted solution.

THE GARLIC ENEMA CAN HELP

Infections
Candida
Colon Cleanse
Diarrhea
Fever Reduction
Fungus
Parasite Removal

GINGER ENEMA

BENEFITS OF GINGER ENEMAS

- Ginger Enemas help reducing gas.
- They are good digestion stimulants.
- Ginger Enemas can help relieve nausea.
- Ginger Enemas ease the symptoms of the cold or flu.
- Ginger Enemas are effective at relieving pain.
- They can help reduce inflammation.
- Ginger Enemas support cardiovascular health.
- They are known for lowering cancer risk.
- Ginger Enemas can relieve sinus and bronchial congestion.
- Ginger Enemas can help stop the bleeding of rectum.
- Ginger Enemas reduce menstrual pain.

PREPARE THE GINGER ENEMA SOLUTION

Ingredients:

1 serving Ginger Extract
Filtered Water

Steps:

1. Boil the water and remove from heat
2. Add Ginger Extract to 2 - 4 cups water
3. Let steep for 15 minutes
4. Heat or cool to warm, comfortable temperature
5. Add the solution to the enema bag or bucket
6. Administer the enema

ADMINISTER THE GINGER ENEMA

The best position to assume when receiving the Ginger Enema is on your back with your hips slightly raised. After the enema has been inserted, roll onto your right side and hold the solution inside for fifteen minutes to 45 minutes before expelling it. Do not roll from side to side.

If you do not feel the urge to expel the liquid, simply stand up and move around as usual until you do. Sometimes the enema will not be evacuated because of poor hydration. The body has absorbed the water and nutrients to its benefit.

THE GINGER ENEMA CAN HELP

Cardiovascular health
Congestion
Digestion
Gas
Inflammation
Menstrual Pain
Nausea

Pain
Rectal Bleeding
Symptoms of the Cold or Flu

GOLDEN ROD ENEMA

BENEFITS OF GOLDEN ROD ENEMAS

- Golden Rod Enemas can help reduce pain.
- Golden Rod Enemas decrease inflammation.
- Golden Rod Enemas act as a diuretic to increase urine flow.
- They can help improve kidney problems.
- Golden Rod Enemas can stop muscle spasms.
- Golden Rod Enemas also treat gout, joint pain and arthritis.
- Golden Rod Enemas treat eczema and other skin conditions.
- Golden Rod Enemas may kill cancer cells.

PREPARE THE GOLDEN ROD ENEMA SOLUTION

Ingredients:

1 serving Golden Rod Extract
Filtered Water

Steps:

1. Heat 2 - 4 cups water to slightly warmer than your body
2. Stir 1 serving Golden Rod Extract into the water
3. Add the solution to the enema bag or bucket
4. Administer the enema

ADMINISTER THE GOLDEN ROD ENEMA

The best position to assume when receiving the Golden Rod Enema is on your back with your hips slightly raised. After the enema has been inserted, roll onto your right side and hold the solution inside for fifteen minutes to 45 minutes before expelling it. Do not roll from side to side.

If you do not feel the urge to expel the liquid, simply stand up and move around as usual until you do. Sometimes the enema will not be evacuated because of poor hydration. The body has absorbed the water and nutrients to its benefit.

THE GOLDEN ROD ENEMA CAN HELP

Arthritis
Cancer
Eczema
Gout
Inflammation
Kidney Problems
Muscle spasms.
Pain
Skin Rejuvenation
Urinary Tract Problems

GREEN BARLEY ENEMA

BENEFITS OF GREEN BARLEY ENEMA

- Green Barley Enemas help repair cellular DNA.
- Green Barley Enemas can improve acne.
- Green Barley Enemas are helpful managing diabetes.
- Green Barley Enemas can help reduce risk of heart disease.
- Green Barley Enemas can reduce high blood pressure.
- They can reduce high cholesterol.
- Green Barley Enemas are used in weight loss protocols.
- Green Barley Enemas contribute to longevity.
- They have anti-aging qualities.
- Green Barley Enemas contribute to increased energy.
- Green Barley Enemas can help improve sleep and reduce insomnia.
- Green Barley Enemas deliver an improved immune response.

PREPARE THE GREEN BARLEY ENEMA SOLUTION

Ingredients:

1 serving Green Barley Powder
Filtered Water

Steps:

1. Heat 2 - 4 cups water to slightly warmer than your body
2. Stir the Green Barley Powder into the water
3. Add the solution to the enema bag or bucket
4. Administer the enema

ADMINISTER THE GREEN BARLEY ENEMA

The best position to assume when receiving the Green Barley Enema is on your back with your hips slightly raised. After the enema has been inserted, roll onto your right side and hold the solution inside for fifteen minutes to 45 minutes before expelling it. Do not roll from side to side.

If you do not feel the urge to expel the liquid, simply stand up and move around as usual until you do. Sometimes the enema will not be evacuated because of poor hydration. The body has absorbed the water and nutrients to its benefit.

THE GREEN BARLEY ENEMA CAN HELP

Acne
Anti-Aging
Diabetes
Heart Disease
High blood Pressure
High cholesterol
Immune Response
Increased Energy

Insomnia
Longevity
Sleep Improvement
Weight Loss

HOPS ENEMA

The Hops Enema is a sedative with therapeutic benefits. Use care with this enema.

BENEFITS OF HOPS ENEMAS

- Hops Enemas are effective in treating insomnia.
- Hops Enemas are known to help diminish hot flashes.
- Hops Enemas protect brain cells from oxidative damage.
- They may slow development of brain disorders.
- Hops Enemas fight against breast, colon, and ovarian cancer cells.

PREPARE THE HOPS ENEMA SOLUTION

Ingredients:

1 serving Hops Powder
Filtered Water

Steps:

1. Heat 2 - 4 cups water to slightly warmer than your body
2. Stir the Hops Powder into the water
3. Add the solution to the enema bag or bucket
4. Administer the enema

ADMINISTER THE HOPS ENEMA

The best position to assume when receiving the Hops Enema is on your back with your hips slightly raised. After the enema has been inserted, roll onto your right side and hold the solution inside for fifteen minutes to 45 minutes before expelling it. Do not roll from side to side.

If you do not feel the urge to expel the liquid, simply stand up and move around as usual until you do. Sometimes the enema will not be evacuated because of poor hydration. The body has absorbed the water and nutrients to its benefit.

CAUTIONS AND CONSIDERATIONS

The Hops Enema may make depression worse. Avoid use.

The Hops Enema contains chemicals that act like estrogen. If you have conditions that are sensitive to hormones you should avoid this enema. Some of these conditions include breast cancer and endometriosis.

The Hops Enema might cause too much sleepiness when combined with anesthesia and other medications during and after surgical procedures. Do not administer 2 weeks before a scheduled surgery or while taking sedatives.

THE HOPS ENEMA CAN HELP

Brain Disorders
Cancer
Hot Flashes
Insomnia
Oxidative Damage

HORSERADISH ENEMA

The Horseradish Enema is rich in vitamins with many health benefits.

BENEFITS OF HORSERADISH ENEMAS

- Horseradish Enemas are used to treat hardening of spleen and liver.
- Horseradish Enemas can help manage the pain of Sciatica.
- Horseradish Enemas ease gout, joint ache.
- Horseradish Enemas can help prevent cancer.
- Horseradish Enemas can slow the spread of cancer.
- Horseradish Enemas strengthen the immune system.
- Horseradish Enemas are useful in treating urinary tract infections.
- They are useful in treating sinus infections.
- Horseradish Enemas. relieve pain and inflammation.
- Horseradish Enemas can help regulate blood pressure.
- Horseradish Enemas aid in digestion.
- Horseradish Enemas can improve the health of your teeth.
- Horseradish Enemas improve your metabolism.
- Horseradish Enemas can help eliminate worms.

PREPARE THE HORSERADISH ENEMA SOLUTION

Ingredients:

1 serving Horseradish Powder
Filtered Water

Steps:

1. Heat 2 - 4 cups water to slightly warmer than your body
2. Stir the Horseradish Powder into the water
3. Add the solution to the enema bag or bucket
4. Administer the enema

ADMINISTER THE HORSERADISH ENEMA

The best position to assume when receiving the Horseradish Enema is on your back with your hips slightly raised. After the enema has been inserted, roll onto your right side and hold the solution inside for fifteen minutes to 45 minutes before expelling it. Do not roll from side to side.

If you do not feel the urge to expel the liquid, simply stand up and move around as usual until you do. Sometimes the enema will not be evacuated because of poor hydration. The body has absorbed the water and nutrients to its benefit.

THE HORSERADISH ENEMA CAN HELP

Blood Pressure
Cancer
Gout
Immune System

Indigestion
Inflammation
Joint Ache
Liver
Metabolism
Sciatica
Sinus Infections
Urinary Tract Infections
Worms

HYDROGEN ENEMA

The Hydrogen Enema is a natural and safe anti-aging remedy that helps brings the body back to homeostasis.

BENEFITS OF HYDROGEN ENEMAS

- Hydrogen Enemas are antioxidant.
- Hydrogen Enemas are anti-inflammatory.
- Hydrogen Enemas may relieve allergies.
- Hydrogen Enemas provide neuroprotective benefits.
- Hydrogen Enemas supports cognitive function.
- Hydrogen Enemas helps reduce fatigue.
- Hydrogen Enemas has anti-aging properties.
- Hydrogen Enemas may help prevent cardiovascular disease.
- Hydrogen Enemas may help with diabetes.
- Hydrogen Enemas may be helpful in neurological disorders.

PREPARE THE HYDROGEN ENEMA SOLUTION

Ingredients:

1 Hydrogen Tablet
Filtered Water

Steps:

1. Heat 2 - 4 cups water to slightly warmer than your body
2. Dissolve the Hydrogen Tablet into the water
3. Add the solution to the enema bag or bucket
4. Administer the enema

ADMINISTER THE HYDROGEN ENEMA

The best position to assume when receiving the Hydrogen Enema is on your back with your hips slightly raised. After the enema has been inserted, roll onto your right side and hold the solution inside for fifteen minutes to 45 minutes before expelling it. Do not roll from side to side.

If you do not feel the urge to expel the liquid, simply stand up and move around as usual until you do. Sometimes the enema will not be evacuated because of poor hydration. The body has absorbed the water and nutrients to its benefit.

THE HYDROGEN ENEMA CAN HELP

Aging
Allergies
Cardiovascular Disease
Cognitive Function
Diabetes
Fatigue
Inflammation
Neurological Disorders

LAVENDER ENEMA

BENEFITS OF LAVENDER ENEMAS

- Lavender Enemas may help improve sleep.
- Lavender Enemas may offer a natural remedy for pain.
- Lavender Enemas reduce blood pressure and heart rate.
- Lavender Enemas could relieve asthma symptoms.
- Lavender Enemas lessens menopausal hot flashes.
- Lavender Enemas help combat fungus growth.
- Lavender Enemas can help with mental health issues.
- Lavender Enemas can help ease headaches.
- Lavender Enemas can reduce nausea.

PREPARE THE LAVENDER ENEMA SOLUTION

Ingredients:

1 serving Lavender Extract
Filtered Water

Steps:

1. Heat 2 - 4 cups water to slightly warmer than your body
2. Stir the Lavender into the water
3. Add the solution to the enema bag or bucket
4. Administer the enema

ADMINISTER THE LAVENDER ENEMA

The best position to assume when receiving the Lavender Enema is on your back with your hips slightly raised. After the enema has been inserted, roll onto your right side and hold the solution inside for fifteen minutes to 45 minutes before expelling it. Do not roll from side to side.

If you do not feel the urge to expel the liquid, simply stand up and move around as usual until you do. Sometimes the enema will not be evacuated because of poor hydration. The body has absorbed the water and nutrients to its benefit.

THE LAVENDER ENEMA CAN HELP

Anxiety
Asthma
Blood Pressure
Depression
Fungus
Headaches
Hot Flashes
Insomnia
Mental Health
Nausea
Pain

LEMON ENEMA

BENEFITS OF LEMON ENEMAS

- Lemon Enemas relieve constipation.
- Lemon Enemas helps balance the pH of your body.
- Lemon Enemas remove biofilm, parasites and mucus from the colon.
- Lemon Enemas may relieve the discomfort of colitis.

PREPARE THE LEMON ENEMA SOLUTION

Ingredients:

Juice of 3 Lemons
Filtered Water

Steps:

1. Heat 2 - 4 cups water to slightly warmer than your body
2. Stir Lemon Juice into the water

3. Add the solution to the enema bag or bucket
4. Administer the enema

ADMINISTER THE LEMON ENEMA

The best position to assume when receiving the Lemon Enema is on your back with your hips slightly raised. After the enema has been inserted, roll onto your right side and hold the solution inside for fifteen minutes to 45 minutes before expelling it. Do not roll from side to side.

If you do not feel the urge to expel the liquid, simply stand up and move around as usual until you do. Sometimes the enema will not be evacuated because of poor hydration. The body has absorbed the water and nutrients to its benefit.

THE LEMON ENEMA CAN HELP

Constipation
pH Imbalance
Parasites
Colitis

MARSHMALLOW ENEMA

BENEFITS OF MARSHMALLOW ENEMAS

- Marshmallow Enemas can reduce mucus in the respiratory tract.
- Marshmallow Enemas can relieve coughs.
- Marshmallow Enemas are soothing for inflamed conditions of bowel.
- Marshmallow Enemas contribute to overall skin health.
- Marshmallow Enemas is effective as a pain reliever.
- Marshmallow Enemas can help repair gut lining.

PREPARE THE MARSHMALLOW ENEMA SOLUTION

Ingredients:

1 serving Marshmallow Extract
Filtered Water

Steps:

1. Heat 2 - 4 cups water to slightly warmer than your body
2. Stir 1 serving Marshmallow Extract into the water
3. Add the solution to the enema bag or bucket
4. Administer the enema

ADMINISTER THE MARSHMALLOW ENEMA

The best position to assume when receiving the Marshmallow Enema is on your back with your hips slightly raised. After the enema has been inserted, roll onto your right side and hold the solution inside for fifteen minutes to 45 minutes before expelling it. Do not roll from side to side.

If you do not feel the urge to expel the liquid, simply stand up and move around as usual until you do. Sometimes the enema will not be evacuated because of poor hydration. The body has absorbed the water and nutrients to its benefit.

CAUTIONS AND CONSIDERATIONS

The Marshmallow Enema has been found to interact with lithium and diabetes drugs. It can also coat the stomach and interfere with absorption of other medications.

THE MARSHMALLOW ENEMA CAN HELP

Coughs
Gut Health
Inflammation
Mucus
Pain
Skin Rejuvenation

MILK AND MOLASSES ENEMA

The Milk and Molasses Enema is known as the M&M Enema. It was used in nursing until it was replaced by more the more convenient pre-made enema formulas.

BENEFITS OF MILK AND MOLASSES ENEMAS

- Milk and Molasses Enemas are efficient in clearing excess or impacted fecal matter from the colon.

PREPARE THE MILK AND MOLASSES ENEMA SOLUTION

Ingredients:

1-2 cups Whole Milk
1-2 cups Blackstrap Molasses

Steps:

1. Warm the milk in a saucepan and bring to a slight boil, do not overheat the milk or it will curdle
2. Remove the pan from the heat
3. Stir in the molasses until the milk and molasses are mixed thoroughly
4. Add the solution to the enema bag or bucket
5. Administer the enema

* Since this is a strong evacuative enema, you do not need much volume for it to be effective. You can use anywhere between 1 and 2 cups each of milk and molasses, but make sure that they are in equal proportion.

ADMINISTER THE MILK AND MOLASSES ENEMA

The best position to assume when receiving the Milk and Molasses is on your back with your hips slightly raised. After the enema has been inserted, roll onto your right side and hold the solution inside for as long as you can. This enema can become uncomfortable. Do not roll from side to side.

CAUTIONS AND CONSIDERATIONS:

The Milk and Molasses Enema is a messy enema. Use a disposable bag or an enema can with replaceable tubing because it is hard to clean the equipment after this enema. You will want to have a thick towel beneath you to soak up any leaks or spills.

The consistency of the Milk and Molasses Enema is much thicker than a water enema. You will need to hang the enema bag much higher than you usually would for a water-based enema to help the solution flow properly.

Administer this type of enema quickly because it can cause discomfort almost immediately, it will be difficult to hold the Milk and Molasses Enema for a long time. For best effects, try to take in the entire amount of enema before you run to the toilet to release your bowels.

THE MILK AND MOLASSES ENEMA CAN HELP

Constipation
Impacted Bowels

MOLASSES ENEMA

Molasses Enemas are very nourishing and a great support of health and well-being.

BENEFITS OF THE MOLASSES ENEMAS

- Molasses Enemas are helpful in treatment of chronic colitis.
- Molasses Enemas increase Iron absorption.
- Molasses Enemas provide relief from menstruation-related problems.
- Molasses Enemas can help control diabetes.
- They can help reduce symptoms of stress.
- Molasses Enemas can be part of cancer treatment.
- Molasses Enemas improve acne and other skin disorders.
- Molasses Enemas provides relief from constipation.
- Molasses Enemas are helpful treating headaches.
- Molasses Enemas counteract anemia.
- Molasses Enemas improve bone and hair health.
- Molasses Enemas help the body maintain electrolyte balance.
- Molasses Enemas contribute to sexual health.
- Molasses Enemas speed wound healing.

- Molasses Enemas strengthen the immune system.
- Molasses Enemas maintain healthy levels of hemoglobin.
- Molasses Enemas improve the formation of new cells in the body.

PREPARE THE MOLASSES ENEMA SOLUTION

Ingredients:

1 serving Organic Molasses
Filtered Water

Steps:

1. Heat 2 - 4 cups water to slightly warmer than your body
2. Stir 1 serving Organic Molasses into the water
3. Add the solution to the enema bag or bucket
4. Administer the enema

ADMINISTER THE MOLASSES ENEMA

The best position to assume when receiving the Molasses Enema is on your back with your hips slightly raised. After the enema has been inserted, roll onto your right side and hold the solution inside for fifteen minutes to 45 minutes before expelling it. Do not roll from side to side.

If you do not feel the urge to expel the liquid, simply stand up and move around as usual until you do. Sometimes the enema will not be evacuated because of poor hydration. The body has absorbed the water and nutrients to its benefit.

THE MOLASSES ENEMA CAN HELP

Anemia
Bone and hair health
Cancer
Cell Growth
Chronic Colitis
Constipation
Diabetes
Electrolyte balance
Headaches
Immune system
Iron Deficiencies
Menstruation Problems
Sexual health
Skin disorders
Stress
Wound Healing

NEEM ENEMA

BENEFITS OF NEEM ENEMAS

- Neem Enemas have excellent antibacterial and antiviral properties.
- Neem Enemas help treat fungus.
- Neem Enemas detoxifies the blood.
- They stimulate the immune system and help fight infections.
- Neem Enemas can reduce candida.
- Neem Enemas can eliminate parasites.
- Neem Enemas can help heal infections of the colon.
- Neem Enemas can be useful in the treatment of ulcerative colitis.
- Neem Enemas can improve skin conditions.

PREPARE THE NEEM ENEMA SOLUTION

Ingredients:

1 Tbsp Neem Leaf Powder
Filtered Water

Steps:

1. Boil the water and remove from heat
2. Add 2 Tbsp Neem Leaf powder to 2 - 4 cups water
3. Let steep for 15 minutes
4. Heat or cool to warm, comfortable temperature
5. Add the solution to the enema bag or bucket
6. Administer the enema

ADMINISTER THE NEEM ENEMA

The best position to assume when receiving the Neem Enema is on your back with your hips slightly raised. After the enema has been inserted, roll onto your right side and hold the solution inside for fifteen minutes to 45 minutes before expelling it. Do not roll from side to side.

If you do not feel the urge to expel the liquid, simply stand up and move around as usual until you do. Sometimes the enema will not be evacuated because of poor hydration. The body has absorbed the water and nutrients to its benefit.

THE NEEM ENEMA CAN HELP

Antibacterial
Antiviral
Blood Purifier
Candida
Colitis
Detoxification
Fungus

Immune System Support
Improved Bowel Functions
Parasites
Skin Rejuvenation

PAU D'ARCO ENEMA

The Pau d'Arco Enema is wonderful for the treatment of internal yeast infections and fungal overgrowth in the colon. It is also helpful in the reduction of parasites. It has powerful antiviral qualities and promotes the ability of the immune system to fight infections. It is a blood purifier and can lessen the symptoms of psoriasis and dermatitis.

BENEFITS OF PAU D'ARCO ENEMAS

The active substances in Pau d'Arco reach the bloodstream faster when taken as an enema than when taken orally. Here are some ways a Pau d'Arco Enema can be helpful.

- Pau d'Arco is a strong antiviral.
- It reduces parasites.
- It is useful in treatment of yeast infections.
- Pau d'Arco is a blood purifier.
- It can lessen the symptoms of psoriasis and dermatitis.
- It strengthens the immune system.

PREPARE THE PAU D'ARCO ENEMA SOLUTION

Ingredients:

1 tsp organic Pau d'Arco Powder
Filtered Water

Steps:

1. Add 1 tsp Pau d'Arco Powder to 2 - 4 cups of boiling water
2. Strain the tea
3. Heat or cool to warm, comfortable temperature
4. Add the solution to the enema bag or bucket
5. Administer the enema

ADMINISTER THE PAU D'ARCO ENEMA

The best position to assume when receiving the Pau d'Arco Enema is on your back with your hips slightly raised. After the enema has been inserted, roll onto your right side and hold the solution inside for fifteen minutes to 45 minutes before expelling it. Do not roll from side to side.

If you do not feel the urge to expel the liquid, simply stand up and move around as usual until you do. Sometimes the enema will not be evacuated because of poor hydration. The body has absorbed the water and nutrients to its benefit.

CAUTIONS AND CONSIDERATIONS:

The use of Pau d'Arco may cause some die-off reactions. If you have a Candida or parasites in the colon, start with a weaker concentration of Pau d'Arco tea in your enema and increase the strength gradually.

THE PAU D'ARCO ENEMA CAN HELP

Anti-Viral
Blood Purifier
Candida
Common Cold
Detoxification
Immune System Support
Improved Circulation
Parasite Removal
Viral Infections
Skin Rejuvenation

PINE BARK ENEMA

The Pine Bark Enema is a super charged retention enema with strong antioxidant, antibacterial, antiviral, anti-carcinogenic, anti-aging, anti-inflammatory and anti-allergic benefits for the body. Pine Bark contains flavonols and bioflavonoids, which have tissue-repairing properties.

BENEFITS OF THE PINE BARK ENEMA

- Pine Bark lowers glucose levels.
- Pine Bark is a natural ear infection remedy and helps prevent hearing loss and improve balance.
- It is a natural remedy and preventive measure for infections.
- It helps reduce hyperpigmentation of human skin while improving the "skin barrier function and extracellular matrix homeostasis."
- Pine Bark helps with erectile dysfunction.
- It scavenges free radicals as a powerful antioxidant.
- Pine Bark helps reduce the inflammation.
- It increases serum NAD+ levels, increasing athletic performance.

- Pine Bark contributes to less cramping and muscle pain.
- It improves blood circulation.
- It improves allergies and asthma.
- It increases the absorption of Vitamin C.

PREPARE THE PINE BARK ENEMA SOLUTION

Ingredients:

2 tsp organic Pine Bark Extract Powder
Filtered Water

Steps:

1. Add 2 Teaspoons Pine Bark Extract Powder to boiling filtered water
2. Simmer over reduced heat for 15 minutes
3. Add water to bring the amount of solution to between 2 - 4 cups
4. Heat or cool to warm, comfortable temperature
5. Add the solution to the enema bag or bucket
6. Administer the enema

ADMINISTER THE PINE BARK ENEMA

The best position to assume when receiving the Pine Bark Enema is on your back with your hips slightly raised. After the enema has been inserted, roll onto your right side and hold the solution inside for fifteen minutes to 45 minutes before expelling it. Do not roll from side to side.

If you do not feel the urge to expel the liquid, simply stand up and move around as usual until you do. Sometimes the enema will not be evacuated because of poor hydration. The body has absorbed the water and nutrients to its benefit.

PINE BARK ENEMA CAN HELP

Allergy Relief
Anti Bacterial
Anti-Inflammatory
Anti-Viral
Asthma
Cancer
Circulation Problems
Common Cold
Congestion
Erectile Dysfunction
Exercise Performance
High Blood Pressure
Hypoglycemia
Immune System Support
Improved Circulation
Prostate Problems
Viral Infections

REISHI MUSHROOM ENEMA

BENEFITS OF REISHI MUSHROOM ENEMAS

- Reishi Mushroom Enemas have cancer-fighting properties.
- Reishi Mushroom Enemas strengthen the immune system response, which is often weakened during chemotherapy.
- Reishi Mushroom Enemas can counteract the effects of aging.
- Reishi Mushroom Enemas may be helpful treating infections.
- Reishi Mushroom Enemas help fight fatigue.
- Reishi Mushroom Enemas may be useful in treatment of depression.

PREPARE THE REISHI MUSHROOM ENEMA SOLUTION

Ingredients:

1 serving Reishi Mushroom Powder
Filtered Water

Steps:

1. Heat 2 - 4 cups water to slightly warmer than your body
2. Stir 1 serving Reishi Mushroom Powder into the water
3. Add the solution to the enema bag or bucket
4. Administer the enema

ADMINISTER THE REISHI MUSHROOM ENEMA

The best position to assume when receiving the Reishi Mushroom Enema is on your back with your hips slightly raised. After the enema has been inserted, roll onto your right side and hold the solution inside for fifteen minutes to 45 minutes before expelling it. Do not roll from side to side.

If you do not feel the urge to expel the liquid, simply stand up and move around as usual until you do. Sometimes the enema will not be evacuated because of poor hydration. The body has absorbed the water and nutrients to its benefit.

THE REISHI MUSHROOM ENEMA CAN HELP

Aging
Cancer
Depression
Fatigue
Immune System
Infections

RESVERATROL ENEMA

BENEFITS OF RESVERATROL ENEMAS

- Resveratrol Enemas help control cholesterol production.
- Resveratrol Enemas may activate genes that resist diseases of aging.
- Resveratrol Enemas protect the brain.
- Resveratrol Enemas have several benefits for diabetes.
- Resveratrol Enemas may help protect against oxidative stress.
- Resveratrol Enemas can help lessen inflammation.
- Resveratrol Enemas help keep blood sugar levels low.
- Resveratrol Enemas strengthens cartilage and ease joint pain.
- Resveratrol Enemas may inhibit cancer cell growth.

PREPARE THE RESVERATROL ENEMA SOLUTION

Ingredients:

1 serving Resveratrol Powder
Filtered Water

Steps:

1. Heat 2 - 4 cups water to slightly warmer than your body
2. Stir 1 serving Resveratrol Powder into the water
3. Add the solution to the enema bag or bucket
4. Administer the enema

ADMINISTER THE RESVERATROL ENEMA

The best position to assume when receiving the Resveratrol Enema is on your back with your hips slightly raised. After the enema has been inserted, roll onto your right side and hold the solution inside for fifteen minutes to 45 minutes before expelling it. Do not roll from side to side.

If you do not feel the urge to expel the liquid, simply stand up and move around as usual until you do. Sometimes the enema will not be evacuated because of poor hydration. The body has absorbed the water and nutrients to its benefit.

THE RESVERATROL ENEMA CAN HELP

Aging
Brain Health
Blood Sugar Levels
Cancer
Cholesterol
Diabetes
Inflammation
Joint Pain
Oxidative Stress

SALT AND SODA ENEMA

BENEFITS OF SALT AND SODA ENEMAS

- The Salt and Soda Enema is helpful to people with excess acidity.
- They help restore the acid-alkaline balance in the body.
- The Salt and Soda Enema prevent and cure ulcers in the colon.

PREPARE THE SALT AND SODA ENEMA SOLUTION

Ingredients:

2 tsp pure Sea Salt
1 Tbsp Baking Soda
Filtered Water

Steps:

1. Heat the filtered water to slightly warmer than your body
2. Add the Sea Salt and Baking Soda to 2 - 4 cups warm water

3. Mix well until the salt and soda are dissolved
4. Add the solution to the enema bag or bucket
5. Administer the enema

ADMINISTER THE SALT AND SODA ENEMA

The best position to assume when receiving the Salt and Soda Enema is on your back with your hips slightly raised. After the enema has been inserted, roll onto your right side and hold the solution inside for fifteen minutes to 45 minutes before expelling it. Do not roll from side to side.

If you do not feel the urge to expel the liquid, simply stand up and move around as usual until you do. Sometimes the enema will not be evacuated because of poor hydration. The body has absorbed the water and nutrients to its benefit.

CAUTION AND CONSIDERATIONS:

Use Salt and Soda Enemas in moderation because regular use of baking soda in enemas may cause too much alkalinity in the body.

THE SALT AND SODA ENEMA CAN HELP

Colitis
Improved Bowel Function
pH Balance

SLIPPERY ELM ENEMA

The Slippery Elm Enema is one of the best treatments to take for any problem in the gastrointestinal tract.

BENEFITS OF SLIPPERY ELM ENEMAS

- Slippery Elm Enemas coats the intestinal wall to aid in healing.
- Slippery Elm Enemas helps relieve intestinal pain and inflammation.
- They help heal hemorrhoids and inflammatory conditions of the bowel.
- They provide relief for constipation and diarrhea.
- Slippery Elm Enemas protect intestinal walls from excess acidity and the formation of ulcers.
- Slippery Elm Enemas are a very rich source of nutrients.
- Slippery Elm Enemas are useful when a person has trouble eating or keeping food down.

PREPARE THE SLIPPERY ELM ENEMA SOLUTION

Ingredients:

2 Tbsp Slippery Elm Powder
Filtered Water

Steps:

1. Boil 2 cups of water and remove from heat
2. 2 Tbsp Slippery Elm Powder
3. Let steep for 5 minutes.
4. Blend the mixture and add up to 1 more quart of water
5. Heat or cool to warm, comfortable temperature
6. Add the solution to the enema bag or bucket
7. Administer the enema

* Do not be tempted to use more of the slippery elm powder in your mixture, slippery elm absorbs a lot of water, and using too much will cause the enema solution to be too thick.

ADMINISTER THE SLIPPERY ELM ENEMA

The best position to assume when receiving the Slippery Elm Enema is on your back with your hips slightly raised. After the enema has been inserted, roll onto your right side and hold the solution inside for fifteen minutes to 45 minutes before expelling it. Do not roll from side to side.

If you do not feel the urge to expel the liquid, simply stand up and move around as usual until you do. Sometimes the enema will not be evacuated because of poor hydration. The body has absorbed the water and nutrients to its benefit.

THE SLIPPERY ELM ENEMA CAN HELP

Intestinal Healing
Intestinal Pain
Inflammation
Hemorrhoids
Inflammatory Bowel Conditions
Constipation
Diarrhea
pH Balance
Ulcers
Nutrition Deficit

SPIRULINA ENEMA

BENEFITS OF SPIRULINA ENEMAS

- Spirulina Enemas can assist the bowels to detox and clean the blood.
- Spirulina Enemas are extremely high in many nutrients.
- Spirulina Enemas are powerful antioxidants.
- Spirulina Enemas are anti-Inflammatory.
- Spirulina Enemas can lower "bad" LDL and triglyceride levels.
- Spirulina Enemas may have anti-cancer properties.
- Spirulina Enemas may help reduce blood pressure.
- Spirulina Enemas can Improves symptoms of allergies.
- Spirulina Enemas may be effective against anemia.
- Spirulina Enemas can improve muscle strength and endurance.
- Spirulina Enemas may help manage blood sugar levels.

PREPARE THE SPIRULINA ENEMA SOLUTION

Ingredients:

1 serving Spirulina Powder
Filtered Water

Steps:

1. Heat 2 - 4 cups water to slightly warmer than your body
2. Stir 1 serving Spirulina Powder into the water
3. Add the solution to the enema bag or bucket
4. Administer the enema

ADMINISTER THE SPIRULINA ENEMA

The best position to assume when receiving the Spirulina Enema is on your back with your hips slightly raised. After the enema has been inserted, roll onto your right side and hold the solution inside for fifteen minutes to 45 minutes before expelling it. Do not roll from side to side.

If you do not feel the urge to expel the liquid, simply stand up and move around as usual until you do. Sometimes the enema will not be evacuated because of poor hydration. The body has absorbed the water and nutrients to its benefit.

THE SPIRULINA ENEMA CAN HELP

Allergies
Anemia
Blood Pressure
Blood Purification
Blood Sugar Levels
Cancer
Cholesterol
Detoxification
Exercise Performance

Inflammation
Nutritional Deficiencies

TURMERIC ENEMA

BENEFITS OF TURMERIC ENEMAS

- Turmeric Enemas are used in effective treatment of Ulcerative colitis.
- Turmeric Enemas are antioxidant.
- Turmeric Enemas support conditions of hypoglycemia
- Turmeric Enemas are a strong anti-inflammatory.
- Turmeric Enemas help manage inflammatory bowel disease.
- Turmeric Enemas may relieve arthritis pain.
- Turmeric Enemas aid in cancer prevention.
- Turmeric Enemas guard cardiovascular health.
- Turmeric Enemas may protect against Alzheimer's disease.
- Turmeric Enemas may help with diabetes.

PREPARE THE TURMERIC ENEMA SOLUTION

Ingredients:

2 Tbsp Organic Turmeric Powder

Filtered Water

Steps:

1. Heat 2 - 4 cups water to slightly warmer than your body
2. Stir 2 Tbsp Organic Turmeric Powder into the water
3. Add the solution to the enema bag or bucket
4. Administer the enema

ADMINISTER THE TURMERIC ENEMA

The best position to assume when receiving the Turmeric Enema is on your back with your hips slightly raised. After the enema has been inserted, roll onto your right side and hold the solution inside for fifteen minutes to 45 minutes before expelling it. Do not roll from side to side.

If you do not feel the urge to expel the liquid, simply stand up and move around as usual until you do. Sometimes the enema will not be evacuated because of poor hydration. The body has absorbed the water and nutrients to its benefit.

THE TURMERIC ENEMA CAN HELP

Alzheimers
Arthritis
Cancer
Cardiovascular Health
Diabetes
Hypoglycemia
Inflammation
Inflammatory Bowel Disease
Ulcerative Colitis

UVA URSI AND HORSETAIL ENEMA

BENEFITS OF UVA URSI AND HORSETAIL ENEMAS

- Uva Ursi and Horsetail Enemas purify the body of toxins and poisons.
- Uva Ursi and Horsetail Enemas can help treat cystitis.
- Uva Ursi and Horsetail Enemas can help clear kidney congestion.
- Uva Ursi and Horsetail Enemas may improve the condition of the skin and nails.
- Uva Ursi and Horsetail Enemas eliminates fluids, contributing to weight loss.
- Uva Ursi and Horsetail Enemas Strengthens our bones and tendons.
- Uva Ursi and Horsetail Enemas reduce bacteria in the urine.
- Uva Ursi and Horsetail Enemas reduce swelling of the bladder and urethra.
- They reduce swelling of the urinary tract.
- Uva Ursi and Horsetail Enemas fight kidney infections.
- Uva Ursi and Horsetail Enemas can soothe the stomach upset.
- Uva Ursi and Horsetail Enemas boost the immune system.

- They reduce inflammation.
- Uva Ursi and Horsetail Enemas help relieve constipation.
- Uva Ursi and Horsetail Enemas are beneficial in treatment of bronchitis.

PREPARE THE UVA URSI AND HORSETAIL ENEMA SOLUTION

Ingredients:

1 serving Uva Ursi Extract
1 serving Horsetail Extract
Filtered Water

Steps:

1. Heat 2 - 4 cups water to slightly warmer than your body
2. Stir 1 serving each of Uva Ursi and Horsetail Extract into the water
3. Add the solution to the enema bag or bucket
4. Administer the enema

ADMINISTER THE UVA URSI AND HORSETAIL ENEMA

The best position to assume when receiving the Uva Ursi Horsetail Enema is on your back with your hips slightly raised. After the enema has been inserted, roll onto your right side and hold the solution inside for fifteen minutes to 45 minutes before expelling it. Do not roll from side to side.

If you do not feel the urge to expel the liquid, simply stand up and move around as usual until you do. Sometimes the enema will not be evacuated because of poor hydration. The body has absorbed the water and nutrients to its benefit.

THE UVA URSI AND HORSETAIL ENEMA CAN HELP

Antibacterial
Bronchitis
Constipation
Cystitis
Detoxification
Fluid Retention
Kidney Congestion
Kidney Infections
Immune System
Inflammation
Skin Rejuvenation
Upset Stomach
Urinary Organ Problems
Weight Loss

UVA URSI ENEMA

BENEFITS OF UVA URSI ENEMAS

- Uva Ursi Enemas reduce bacteria in the urine.
- Uva Ursi Enemas reduce swelling of the bladder and urethra.
- They reduce swelling of the urinary tract.
- Uva Ursi Enemas fight kidney infections.
- Uva Ursi Enemas can soothe the stomach upset.
- Uva Ursi Enemas boost the immune system.
- They reduce inflammation.
- Uva Ursi Enemas are helpful detoxifying the body
- Uva Ursi Enemas help relieve constipation.
- Uva Ursi Enemas are beneficial in treatment of bronchitis.

PREPARE THE UVA URSI ENEMA SOLUTION

Ingredients:

1 serving Uva Ursi Extract
Filtered Water

Steps:

1. Heat 2 - 4 cups water to slightly warmer than your body
2. Stir 1 serving Uva Ursi Extract into the water
3. Add the solution to the enema bag or bucket
4. Administer the enema

ADMINISTER THE UVA URSI ENEMA

The best position to assume when receiving the Uva Ursi Enema is on your back with your hips slightly raised. After the enema has been inserted, roll onto your right side and hold the solution inside for fifteen minutes to 45 minutes before expelling it. Do not roll from side to side.

If you do not feel the urge to expel the liquid, simply stand up and move around as usual until you do. Sometimes the enema will not be evacuated because of poor hydration. The body has absorbed the water and nutrients to its benefit.

THE UVA URSI ENEMA CAN HELP

Antibacterial
Bronchitis
Constipation
Detoxification
Kidney Infections
Immune System
Inflammation
Upset Stomach
Urinary Organ Problems

VALERIAN ENEMA

BENEFITS OF VALERIAN ENEMAS

- Valerian Enemas reduce symptoms of anxiety.
- Valerian Enemas are sedative and encourage sleep.
- Valerian Enemas can reduce flatulence.
- Valerian Enemas can help reduce hot flashes.

PREPARE THE VALERIAN ENEMA SOLUTION

Ingredients:

1 serving Valerian Extract
Filtered Water

Steps:

1. Heat 2 - 4 cups water to slightly warmer than your body
2. Stir 1 serving Valerian Extract into the water

3. Add the solution to the enema bag or bucket
4. Administer the enema

ADMINISTER THE VALERIAN ENEMA

The best position to assume when receiving the Valerian Enema is on your back with your hips slightly raised. After the enema has been inserted, roll onto your right side and hold the solution inside for fifteen minutes to 45 minutes before expelling it. Do not roll from side to side.

If you do not feel the urge to expel the liquid, simply stand up and move around as usual until you do. Sometimes the enema will not be evacuated because of poor hydration. The body has absorbed the water and nutrients to its benefit.

CAUTIONS AND CONSIDERATIONS

Do not use a Valerian Enema and call your doctor immediately if you have signs of liver impairment including persistent fatigue, nausea, vomiting, dark urine, clay-colored stools or jaundice.

The Valerian Enema may cause excessive sleepiness if combined with alcohol, sedatives, some antidepressants, over-the-counter sleeping pills, or cold and flu remedies containing codeine, diphenhydramine, or doxylamine.

Due to the lack of safety research, The Valerian Enema should not be used in children, pregnant women, or nursing mothers. It should also be used with extreme caution in heavy drinkers or people with liver disease.

THE VALERIAN ENEMA CAN HELP

Anxiety

Flatulence
Hot Flashes
Insomnia

YARROW ENEMA

BENEFITS OF YARROW ENEMAS

- The Yarrow Enema induces perspiration and is good for fever reduction.
- They soothe and heal mucus membranes.
- They help loosen and flush mucus from intestines.
- They reduce inflammation of the abdomen and intestines.
- They are help in treating hemorrhoids, diarrhea and gas.

PREPARE THE YARROW ENEMA SOLUTION

Ingredients:

2 Tbsp dried Yarrow
Filtered Water

Steps:

1. Boil the water and remove from heat

2. Add 2 Tbsp Yarrow to 2 - 4 cups water
3. Let steep for 15 minutes
4. Heat or cool to warm, comfortable temperature
5. Add the solution to the enema bag or bucket
6. Administer the enema

ADMINISTER THE YARROW ENEMA

The best position to assume when receiving the Yarrow Enema is on your back with your hips slightly raised. After the enema has been inserted, roll onto your right side and hold the solution inside for fifteen minutes to 45 minutes before expelling it. Do not roll from side to side.

If you do not feel the urge to expel the liquid, simply stand up and move around as usual until you do. Sometimes the enema will not be evacuated because of poor hydration. The body has absorbed the water and nutrients to its benefit.

CAUTIONS AND CONSIDERATIONS

Yarrow contains salicylic acid. If you have a known allergy to aspirin, which has a high concentration of salicylic acid, do not administer the Yarrow Enema.

THE YARROW ENEMA CAN HELP

Bowel Functions
Diarrhea
Fever
Hemorrhoids
Inflammation

IMPLANT ENEMAS

An Implant Enema is made with a smaller amount of liquid, often only one cup and is retained permanently. This is a beneficial way to introduce probiotics and minerals to the system. A great strategy for taking an Implant Enema is to administer right before going to sleep.

ADMINISTER THE IMPLANT ENEMA

The best position to assume when receiving the Implant Enema Implant is on your back with your hips slightly raised. After the enema has been inserted, roll onto your right side and hold the liquid inside up to 45 minutes before releasing it. Do not roll from side to side.

Some people claim benefits to holding the liquids long enough for them to be fully absorbed by the body. This is easily achieved by administering the Implant Enema Implant before going to sleep.

HEALTH NOTE

All information in this enema collection is purely for research and informational purposes only. Follow any of these cleansing protocol procedures at your own risk.

ACIDOPHILUS ENEMA

BENEFITS OF ACIDOPHILUS ENEMA

- Acidophilus Implant Enemas help replace the friendly bacteria in the colon.
- Acidophilus Implant Enemas contribute to a healthy gut.
- Acidophilus Implant Enemas can eliminate constipation.

PREPARATION OF ACIDOPHILUS ENEMA SOLUTION

Ingredients:

1/8 Tsp Acidophilus Powder
Filtered Water

Steps:

1. Heat 1 - 2 cups water to slightly warmer than your body
2. Stir 1/8 teaspoon of Acidophilus Powder to the water
3. Add the solution to the enema bag or bucket

4. Administer the enema

ADMINISTER THE ACIDOPHILUS ENEMA

The best position to assume when receiving the Acidophilus Enema Implant is on your back with your hips slightly raised. After the enema has been inserted, roll onto your right side and hold the liquid inside up to 45 minutes before releasing it. Do not roll from side to side.

Some people claim benefits to holding the liquids long enough for them to be fully absorbed by the body. This is easily achieved by administering the Acidophilus Enema Implant before going to sleep.

THE ACIDOPHILUS ENEMA CAN HELP

Constipation
Gut Bacteria Balance
Leaky Gut Syndrome

CBD ENEMA

BENEFITS OF CBD ENEMAS

- CBD Enemas are an effective pain reliever.
- CBD Enemas can relieve menstrual cramps .
- CBD Enemas can reduce hemorrhoid inflammation.
- CBD Enemas can relieve lower back pain.
- CBD Enemas can relieve Sciatica.
- CBD Enemas can help with Irritable Bowel Syndrome.
- CBD Enemas could reduce anxiety and depression.
- CBD Enemas may help reduce symptoms related to cancer and side effects related to cancer treatment, like nausea, vomiting and pain.
- CBD Enemas are helpful treating neurological disorders like epilepsy and multiple sclerosis.
- CBD Enemas could benefit heart health.
- CBD Enemas has anti-tumor effects.

*Note: While most people report full body effects of the CBD Enema there are some who will experience more localized benefits such as pain relief near the pelvic area, etc.

PREPARE THE CBD ENEMA SOLUTION

Ingredients:

500+ MG Organic CBD or Hemp Oil
Filtered Water

Steps:

1. Heat 2 - 4 cups water to slightly warmer than your body
2. Add 500+ MG Organic CBD or Hemp Oil to the water
3. Add the solution to the enema bag or bucket
4. Administer the enema

ADMINISTER THE CBD ENEMA

The best position to assume when receiving the CBD Enema Implant is on your back with your hips slightly raised. After the enema has been inserted, roll onto your right side and hold the liquid inside up to 45 minutes before releasing it. Do not roll from side to side.

Some people claim benefits to holding the liquids long enough for them to be fully absorbed by the body. This is easily achieved by administering the Probiotic Enema Implant before going to sleep.

THE CBD ENEMA CAN HELP

Pain
Anxiety
Back Pain
Cancer
Depression
Epilepsy

Heart Health
Hemorrhoids
Inflammation
Irritable Bowel Syndrome
Menstrual Cramps
Multiple Sclerosis
Neurological Disorders
Sciatica
Tumors

COCONUT OIL ENEMA

BENEFITS OF COCONUT OIL ENEMAS

- Coconut Oil Enemas can kill harmful microorganisms.
- Coconut Oil Enemas help kill the bacterias Staphylococcus and Candida.
- Coconut Oil Enemas may help reduce seizures.
- Coconut Oil Enemas can raise the good HDL cholesterol.
- Coconut Oil Enemas may boost brain function in Alzheimer's patients.
- Coconut Oil Enemas can help burn fat, especially harmful abdominal fat.
- Coconut Oil Enemas has anti-fungal, antibacterial and anti-viral properties.
- Coconut Oil Enemas reduces inflammation.

PREPARE THE COCONUT OIL ENEMA SOLUTION

Ingredients:

1 serving Organic Coconut Oil
Filtered Water

Steps:

1. Heat 1 - 2 cups water to slightly warmer than your body
2. Stir 1 serving Organic Coconut Oil into the water
3. Add the solution to the enema bag or bucket
4. Administer the enema

ADMINISTER THE COCONUT OIL ENEMA

The best position to assume when receiving the Coconut Oil Enema Implant is on your back with your hips slightly raised. Use an Enema Bulb Syringe to administer a Coconut Oil Enema. After the enema has been inserted, roll onto your right side and hold the liquid inside for 15 to 45 minutes before releasing it. Do not roll from side to side.

Some people claim benefits to holding the liquids long enough for them to be fully absorbed by the body. This is easily achieved by administering the Coconut Oil Enema Implant before going to sleep.

It's a good idea to follow a Coconut Oil Enema with a Gentle Cleansing Enema. This will help remove all the traces of oil and prevent leaking oil later.

CAUTIONS AND CONSIDERATIONS

Choose organic, virgin coconut oil In order to get the best health benefits from the Coconut Oil Enema. Refined oils may contain impurities you will not want to place inside your body.

THE COCONUT OIL ENEMA CAN HELP

Alzheimers
Antibacterial

Antiviral
Cognitive Function
Cholesterol
Fungus
Inflammation
Seizures
Weight Loss

ECHINACEA ENEMA

BENEFITS OF ECHINACEA ENEMAS

- Echinacea Enemas are good antioxidants.
- Echinacea Enemas are antiseptic, antibacterial, and antiviral.
- Echinacea Enemas help treatment of upper respiratory tract infections.
- Echinacea Enemas are effective blood cleansers.
- They are helpful in skin conditions like acne, eczema and boils.
- Echinacea Enemas protect abdominal organs against peritonitis.

PREPARE THE ECHINACEA ENEMA SOLUTION

Ingredients:

1 Dose Echinacea Extract
Filtered Water

Steps:

1. Heat 1 - 2 cups water to slightly warmer than your body
2. Stir 1 dose of Echinacea Extract into the water
3. Add the solution to the enema bag or bucket
4. Administer the enema

ADMINISTER THE ECHINACEA ENEMA

The best position to assume when receiving the Echinacea Enema Implant is on your back with your hips slightly raised. After the enema has been inserted, roll onto your right side and hold the liquid inside up to 45 minutes before releasing it. Do not roll from side to side.

Some people claim benefits to holding the liquids long enough for them to be fully absorbed by the body. This is easily achieved by administering the Echinacea Enema Implant before going to sleep.

THE ECHINACEA ENEMA CAN HELP

Antibacterial
Antiviral
Blood Purification
Inflammation
Peritonitis
Skin Rejuvenation
Upper Respiratory Tract Infections

MTC ENEMA

BENEFITS OF MTC ENEMAS

- MCT Enemas increases the release of two hormones that decrease hunger.
- MCT Enemas are a source of energy.
- MCT Enemas can fuel the brain.
- MCT Enemas may reduce lactate buildup and help use fat for energy.
- MCT Enemas may help manage Epilepsy, Alzheimer's Disease and Autism.
- MCT Enemas may reduce risk factors for heart disease.
- MCT Enemas can help control blood sugar levels.
- MCT Enemas can help manage Diabetes.

PREPARE THE MTC ENEMA SOLUTION

Ingredients:

1 serving Organic MCT Oil

Filtered Water

Steps:

1. Heat 1 - 2 cups water to slightly warmer than your body
2. Stir 1 serving Organic MCT Oil into the water
3. Add the solution to the enema bag or bucket
4. Administer the enema

ADMINISTER THE MTC ENEMA

The best position to assume when receiving the MTC Enema Implant is on your back with your hips slightly raised. If you use MCT Oil then use an Enema Bulb Syringe to administer the enema. After the enema has been inserted, roll onto your right side and hold the liquid inside for 15 to 45 minutes before releasing it. Do not roll from side to side.

Some people claim benefits to holding the liquids long enough for them to be fully absorbed by the body. This is easily achieved by administering the MCT Enema Implant before going to sleep.

It's a good idea to follow a MCT Oil Enema with a Gentle Cleansing Enema. This will help remove all the traces of oil and prevent leaking oil later.

CAUTIONS AND CONSIDERATIONS

High doses of MCT oil may increase the amount of fat in your liver in the long term. Use the MCT Enema carefully.

THE MTC ENEMA CAN HELP

Alzheimer's Disease
Autism
Blood Sugar Levels
Brain Function

Decrease Hunger
Diabetes
Energy
Epilepsy
Heart Disease
Metabolism

MINERAL ENEMA

BENEFITS OF MINERAL ENEMAS

- Mineral Enemas provide support to the adrenals.
- Mineral Enemas support a healthy thyroid.
- Mineral Enemas contribute to increased energy and well-being.
- Mineral Enemas replace deficient minerals.

PREPARE THE MINERAL ENEMA IMPLANT

Ingredients:

1 Dose / Serving Mineral Supplement Powder
Filtered Water

Steps:

1. Heat 1 - 2 cups water to slightly warmer than your body
2. Stir 1 dose of Mineral Supplement Powder into the water

3. Add the solution to the enema bag or bucket
4. Administer the enema

ADMINISTER THE MINERAL ENEMA

The best position to assume when receiving the Mineral Enema Implant is on your back with your hips slightly raised. After the enema has been inserted, roll onto your right side and hold the liquid inside up to 45 minutes before releasing it. Do not roll from side to side.

Some people claim benefits to holding the liquids long enough for them to be fully absorbed by the body. This is easily achieved by administering the Mineral Enema Implant before going to sleep.

THE MINERAL ENEMA CAN HELP

Adrenal Support
Increased Energy
Mineral Deficiencies
Thyroid Support

NAD+ BOOSTER ENEMA

NAD+ Booster Enemas may switch "off" the aging genes and some compare NAD to the fountain of youth.

BENEFITS OF NAD+ BOOSTER ENEMAS

- NAD+ Booster Enemas activate enzymes that promote healthy aging.
- NAD+ Booster Enemas may extend life span.
- NAD+ Booster Enemas may increase endurance.
- NAD+ Booster Enemas may improve cognitive function.
- They can enhances cellular energy.
- They help converting food into energy.
- NAD+ Booster Enemas in the repairing of damaged DNA.
- NAD+ Booster Enemas fortify cell defense systems.
- NAD+ Booster Enemas help set the body's internal clock or circadian rhythm.
- They can help treat jet lag.
- NAD+ Booster Enemas may help protect brain cells.
- NAD+ Booster Enemas may lower the risk of heart disease.
- NAD+ Booster Enemas may contribute to weight loss.

- NAD+ Booster Enemas may lower the risk of cancer.

PREPARE THE NAD+ BOOSTER ENEMA SOLUTION

Ingredients:

2 capsules NAD+
Filtered Water

Steps:

1. Heat 1 - 2 cups water to slightly warmer than your body
2. Dissolve the powder from 2 capsules NAD+ into the water
3. Add the solution to the enema bag or bucket
4. Administer the enema

ADMINISTER THE NAD+ BOOSTER ENEMA

The best position to assume when receiving the NAD+ Booster Enema Implant is on your back with your hips slightly raised. After the enema has been inserted, roll onto your right side and hold the liquid inside up to 45 minutes before releasing it. Do not roll from side to side.

Some people claim benefits to holding the liquids long enough for them to be fully absorbed by the body. This is easily achieved by administering the NAD+ Booster Enema Implant before going to sleep.

THE NAD+ BOOSTER ENEMA CAN HELP

Aging
Brain Health
Cancer

Cell Health
Cellular Energy
Circadian Rhythm
Cognitive Function
Endurance
Heart Disease
Jet Lag
Longevity
Metabolism
Weight Loss

PROBIOTIC ENEMA

A Probiotic Enema Implant is recommended for those who administer Coffee Enemas and other enemas on a regular basis. It help replenish and protect the gut bacteria. It is also indicated for candida and other yeast infections.

BENEFITS OF PROBIOTIC ENEMAS

- Probiotic Enemas can improve your overall gut health.
- Probiotic Enemas can fight agains Candida.
- Probiotic Enemas bypass stomach acids that kill 60% of the probiotics by placing them directly in the colon.
- Probiotic Enemas have led to increased metabolism.
- Probiotic Enemas contribute to weight loss.
- Probiotic Enemas help improve immune system function.
- Probiotic Enemas help with diarrhea, constipation and bloating.

PREPARE THE PROBIOTIC ENEMA SOLUTION

Ingredients:

1 Serving Probiotic Powder
Filtered Water

Steps:

1. Heat 1 - 2 cups water to slightly warmer than your body
2. Add 1 Serving Probiotic Powder to the water
3. Add the solution to the enema bag or bucket
4. Administer the enema

ADMINISTER THE PROBIOTIC ENEMA

The best position to assume when receiving the Probiotic Enema Implant is on your back with your hips slightly raised. After the enema has been inserted, roll onto your right side and hold the liquid inside up to 45 minutes before releasing it. Do not roll from side to side.

Some people claim benefits to holding the liquids long enough for them to be fully absorbed by the body. This is easily achieved by administering the Probiotic Enema Implant before going to sleep.

CAUTIONS AND CONSIDERATIONS

Probiotic Enemas are usually beneficial but they can lead to infections in people with compromised immune systems.

THE PROBIOTIC ENEMA CAN HELP

Absorption
Bloating

Candida
Constipation
Diarrhea
Gut Health
Immune System
Metabolism
Weight Loss

TMG ENEMA

The TMG Enema is a powerful enema offering the benefits of trimethylglycine.

BENEFITS OF TMG ENEMAS

- TMG Enemas helps with toxic metal removal.
- TMG Enemas aids protein synthesis in the body.
- TMG Enemas promote a positive mood and emotional balance.
- TMG Enemas help prevent homocysteine adverse effects.
- TMG Enemas support numerous brain and other organ functions.
- TMG Enemas may protect the heart.
- TMG Enemas help cells adapt to stress.
- TMG Enemas may protect against premature programmed cell death (apoptosis).
- TMG Enemas keeps cells hydrated and increases stress resilience.
- TMG Enemas may increase blood levels of nitric oxide which widens blood vessels and increases muscle blood flow .

- TMG Enemas can improve exercise performance by increasing nutrient delivery and waste excretion.
- TMG Enemas may contribute to better reaction time, memory, and brain function.
- TMG Enemas may improve cognitive function.
- TMG Enemas may help protect the liver.

PREPARE THE TMG ENEMA SOLUTION

Ingredients:

1 serving TMG Powder
Filtered Water

Steps:

1. Heat 1 - 2 cups water to slightly warmer than your body
2. Stir 1 serving TMG Powder into the water
3. Add the solution to the enema bag or bucket
4. Administer the enema

ADMINISTER THE TMG ENEMA

The best position to assume when receiving the TMG Enema Implant is on your back with your hips slightly raised. After the enema has been inserted, roll onto your right side and hold the liquid inside up to 45 minutes before releasing it. Do not roll from side to side.

Some people claim benefits to holding the liquids long enough for them to be fully absorbed by the body. This is easily achieved by administering the TMG Enema Implant before going to sleep.

THE TMG ENEMA CAN HELP

Brain Health
Cellular Health
Circulation
Cognitive Function
Detoxification
Emotional Well-being
Exercise Performance
Heart Health
Liver
Protein Synthesis

VITAMIN E ENEMA

BENEFITS OF VITAMIN E ENEMAS

- Vitamin E Enemas may prevent coronary heart disease.
- Vitamin E Enemas support immune function.
- Vitamin E Enemas can prevent inflammation.
- Vitamin E Enemas may promote eye health.
- Vitamin E Enemas can lower the risk of cancer.

PREPARE THE VITAMIN E ENEMA SOLUTION

Ingredients:

1 serving Vitamin E Oil
Filtered Water

Steps:

1. Heat 1 - 2 cups water to slightly warmer than your body
2. Stir 1 serving Vitamin E Oil into the water

3. Add the solution to the enema bag or bucket
4. Administer the enema

ADMINISTER THE VITAMIN E ENEMA

The best position to assume when receiving the Vitamin E Enema Implant is on your back with your hips slightly raised. After the enema has been inserted, roll onto your right side and hold the liquid inside up to 45 minutes before releasing it. Do not roll from side to side.

Some people claim benefits to holding the liquids long enough for them to be fully absorbed by the body. This is easily achieved by administering the Vitamin E Enema Implant before going to sleep.

CAUTIONS AND CONSIDERATIONS

Vitamin E oil is a supplement and a beauty product and is not regulated. This means that two vitamin E oils might be different concentrations and produce different effects in the same person.

Many Vitamin E products contain additional ingredients. It is important to read the label and buy the purest product to insert with the Vitamin E Enema.

THE VITAMIN E ENEMA CAN HELP

Cancer
Heart Disease
Immune System
Inflammation
Vision

CAUTIONS AND CONSIDERATIONS

Regular use of Healing Enemas are safe and promote health and well-being with regular use. But there are cautions that must be considered for a successful enema application.

CLEANLINESS

Infections associated with enemas can be avoided by following guidelines for cleanliness.

It is important to keep the area where the enema is taken is clean. Use clean towels or mats to lie on. Spray the area and equipment with Hydrogen Peroxide and a solution of Castile soap. Do not use bleach because it will introduce poison into your body. Clean the equipment thoroughly and store it in a clean place. Clean any spills on the toilet and the sink. Use paper towels to clean spills and equipment.

Clean everything!

INJURY

Injuries associated with enemas can be avoided by following some safety guidelines.

Always use a lubricant. Castor Oil and Coconut Oil are the preferred choices. Do not use Vaseline or Mineral Oils as they are by-products of petroleum processing and are toxic.

Insert the enema tip slowly. Tears in the colon are a result of rough handling and are dangerous. If the insertion becomes painful, stop.

Make sure you check the temperature of the enema solution before you apply it. I should be slightly warm to the touch - between 100 and 104 degrees Fahrenheit.

AVOID TOXINS AND POISONS

- Use filtered water because tap water contains chlorine and other additives.
- Use glass jars because plastics release toxins.
- Bleach is poison to living things, including you.
- Use organic and non-GMO ingredients to avoid putting chemicals into your body.

CONSIDER THE BENEFITS

As you use enemas as part of your health routine you will notice a lightness and clarity that some people have described as a euphoria. Focus on the good feelings of improved health and self care. Your positive mindset towards enemas will help you relax and experince success and all the benefits of the enema of your choice.

FOR YOUR INFORMATION

The content of The Healing Enema Cookbook is does not equal medical advice.

The information in this book is not meant to diagnose, treat or cure any illness, sickness or disease. Please consult your physician before you try any of these cleansing protocols. All information in this enema collection is purely for research and informational purposes only. Follow any of these cleansing protocol procedures at your own risk.

There are many practices, including Healing Enemas, that one can do to maintain, improve, and treat their own health. There are times when medical advice and treatment should be pursued. Please use your judgement in this wisely.

Links to recommended products are for your reference and convenience. Some links will provide additional income to support this book.

Here's to your health!

Made in the USA
Columbia, SC
17 June 2022